JUST IN TIME

María Laura Sánchez Puerta

JUST IN TIME

by María Laura Sánchez Puerta

Published by María Laura Sánchez Puerta

Cover photo by María Laura Sánchez Puerta

ISBN: 978-1-7376730-2-6
Library of Congress Control Number: 2023914544
First Edition

To our families

(. . .) And thus, when later comes looking for me
Who knows what death, anxiety of the living
Who knows what loneliness, end of all lovers
I can tell myself of the love (that I had):
May it not be immortal, since it is flame,
But may it be infinite while it lasts.

(Vinicius de Moraes, *Sonnet of Fidelity*)

Chapters

Morgan	1
The Guy from Match.com	3
The Decision	11
A Family	21
California Boy	43
From South to North	51
The Word I Cannot Pronounce	75
The Time of Uneasiness	97
Husband & Wife	113
On That Day	133
Another Life	151

Morgan

I remember exactly.

The barefoot late-January walk along the beach of Monte Hermoso, where I spent so many summers of my life. The Recalada Lighthouse. The green color of the sea as it curls. The clouds on the horizon calm and companionable, as if they are telling me: "You didn't choose this new life, but everything will be all right. Everything *has to* be all right." As if he is in these clouds, in this immensity, and I can feel his company. I stop by the lighthouse, and in its red and white metal structure see a sentinel watching over me and mine at this moment.

And I write, like an incantation, his name in the sand: Morgan.

CHAPTER ONE

The Guy from Match.com

"Come on, Laura! We need to use the bathroom! Come on out!"

They knocked on the door for the tenth time, laughing. I stifled my own laughter. I'd been locked with the phone in the bathroom of a friend's house for an hour. Now a group was glued to the door trying to listen in on my conversation, as if we were a bunch of teenagers and not sophisticated, proper thirty-somethings.

After a dozen emails back and forth, Morgan had finally called me, and I liked his voice. I couldn't find any better place than the bathroom to escape my gaggle of friends and talk quietly with him. It wasn't the most elegant thing in the world, but at least I had some privacy! Not a lot, though.

"So, has he asked you out yet? Go for it, Laura!" my friends shouted from outside.

No, he hadn't asked me out yet.

"I'm going on a three-week trip on Friday," I told Morgan.

I had already mentioned it to him in one of my emails: the World Bank was sending me on a work assignment to Peru and Bolivia for two weeks, and the third I would spend in Argentina visiting my family. But my reminder worked.

"Let's go for a coffee before your trip," he proposed.

We made a date for the following Friday, September 5, 6:00p.m., at the Starbucks on Clarendon Boulevard, near Washington, DC's Rosslyn station.

I was eager to meet him in person. But somehow, especially after this conversation, which flowed so lightly, his voice so calm, I felt like I already knew him.

I could feel my friends' excitement on the other side of the door: "It's a date!"

* * *

That summer of 2008, it had been a year since I decided to break off the long-distance relationship I had sustained as long as I could with a Colombian boyfriend. With me settled in Washington, DC, since I had finished my PhD in 2005, and him in Bogota without plans to move to the US, our relationship was frayed. I was worn out.

A year after we broke up for good, back from a month-long trip to Morocco to perfect my French, I was really looking forward to meeting someone. To having a good time, yes, but also to finding a person with whom I could have a close, real bond, someone with whom I could plan a whole life. But where to meet that someone? My job as a labor economist for the World Bank had me travelling all the time, and those trips weren't exactly ideal for meeting anyone. I lived in a city with a large majority of women and a lot of married men.

When my friend Kiran first offered to help me set up a profile on the relationship site Match.com, I said no. But then I thought better of it: I've always been very proactive, so why not?

At the time I was having life coaching sessions in addition to traditional therapy with a psychologist. I was trying to set and achieve goals to increase my well-being in as many dimensions as I could. I trained for and ran a 10K race as part of a fundraiser for a friend's NGO that provides free legal services to vulnerable women in the DC area. And I realized a profile on this website would also be a push in the right direction.

So I looked for my best recent photo, from a wedding. In it I am looking at the camera and smiling, with perfectly straight hair and a lamé dress that rides the line between elegance and sensuality. Done. All that was left was to write the profile, with my characteristics and the ones I was looking for in my date. And then to see what happened.

Match.com		
In my own words	I was born in Argentina. I came to Ithaca, USA, to do my graduate studies (I loved every moment of those years, especially the atmosphere of the town and the waterfalls inside the campus). I moved to DC three years ago to work in international development. Passionate about tennis, languages and travel.	
My interests	Camping. Coffee and conversation. Movies. Playing sports. Traveling and touring. Volunteering.	
Sport and exercise	I train 3-4 times a week. Biking, dancing, skiing, tennis, walking/hiking.	
Pets	I like birds, dogs and horses.	
Political views	Liberal	
Sign	Aries	
	Me	My date
Height	5′8″	5′4″ to 6′10″
Body type	Athletic and toned	Average type
Eyes	Brown	I have no preference
Hair	Dark brown	I have no preference
Smoker	No way	No way
Drinker	Social drinker	Social drinker or no drinker
Occupation	International Development	I have no preference
Income	No answer	I have no preference
Marital Status	Single	Single
Children	No	No
Have children someday	Someday	Definitely someday
Ethnicity	Latino/Hispanic	I have no preference
Religion	Spiritual but not religious	I have no preference
Languages	English, French, Spanish, German	English
Education	PhD/Postdoctorate	Graduate/PhD/Postdoctorate

The messages started coming in . . . all kinds of strange messages. I didn't have many strong preferences, but no man who contacted me met *any* of my requirements! So I decided to look for myself, searching a geographical range close to my home in Arlington. That didn't narrow it down either, until I found the key word: tennis, my passion since I was a child. I had even played in national tournaments in Argentina. If there was another tennis enthusiast like me on that dating site, I wanted to find him.

There were only three men whose profiles included the word "tennis." I wrote to the two I liked. One didn't respond. I immediately received a message from the other, someone who used the handle *ghostwriter24* and in his profile defined himself as "crazy about tennis":

> Thanks for contacting me! Do you play tennis? I went to the US Open yesterday. I saw a lot of very good players from Argentina. Del Potro is one of the best in the tournament, I think he can win it. What did you study at Cornell? I didn't know there were waterfalls on campus, sounds great. Do you speak any languages besides Spanish and English?
>
> Take care, Morgan

Within just a week on Match.com, I had found a man I liked. I liked his relaxed tone and his profile picture showing a serious guy with glasses and a sweet smile posing in front of a bridge on a trip to Europe. He looked quiet, but adventurous. Five eleven, dark haired, 187 pounds. He was single, Jewish but not practicing, wanted to have children (two!) someday, did not smoke, was athletic, and only drank at social gatherings. He defined himself as curious, a reader, easy-going, passionate about politics, science, history, and cinema. I replied. The messages started flowing back and forth.

Morgan had been born and raised in California and had just returned from a family party there celebrating his 40th birthday. He had come to Washington, DC, from Cincinnati, Ohio, in 2005, the same year I did. He lived close to me. He knew a lot about tennis. He didn't seem to be in any hurry about asking me out to dinner right away. But he did seem to be serious. Something about him—or maybe my sixth sense—told me so.

That Friday, the day before I left for my trip to South America, I was on time for our meeting at the café on Clarendon Boulevard. I recognized Morgan right away. He was already seated, waiting for me. Three hours later, the Starbucks closed and we were still talking: about the US Open, about our jobs. About my life in Bahía Blanca. About his childhood in California. About our families and how important they were to both of us. We talked as if we had known each other all our lives. I liked everything he had written in his emails, I liked his picture on Match.com and now I liked it when we talked. In my mind it was all *check, check, check.*

It started to rain.

"I'll drive you home," he said.

I didn't hesitate in getting into his car. He dropped me off at my front door. I knew he was as happy as I was with our date. I knew that we had both realized we had a lot in common. I knew that I was going to see him again. And I knew that, as soon as I walked into my house, I was going to Google a phrase from our conversation that I had purposely retained in my memory: myxopapillary ependymoma.

CHAPTER TWO

The Decision

"Myxopapillary ependymomas are slow-growing tumors of the spine. They can be external or internal, postsacral or presacral."

"They are known to recur even after complete removal."

"Internal ones can spread through the nervous system but rarely metastasize further, while external ones do have a significant risk of spreading."

"The lungs are the most common site of metastasis, although it is also known in the liver, bone and lymphatic system."

"The treatment is total removal, which makes cure possible without external therapy."

"Radiation has not been adequately studied in these cases."

"Partial excision has a high chance of recurrence."

"Chemotherapy has not proven to be beneficial."

"Patients with total excision have a good prognosis, with a median survival of nineteen years."

"If metastases develop, survival in this type of ependymoma is unlikely."

"When the tumor recurs, survival is unlikely after five years."

The sentences from the most serious medical websites I found that night piled up before my eyes. I decided to send my sister, a biologist, all the papers I could find on the subject to help me understand. Myxopapillary ependymoma—external, internal, presacral, postsacral? I didn't know. But that was the disease Morgan had suffered from. And he had told me about it on our first date.

*   *   *

He told me in the same natural way he talked about his travels, his love of the outdoors, or his work as a tax attorney for a federal government agency. Since his early twenties Morgan had suffered from a lot of back pain. After countless ineffectual visits to chiropractors and doctors—they thought it was something muscular—an MRI revealed in 2007 that the pain was the result of a "grapefruit-sized" tumor in his spine.

Since it is sometimes possible to remove it completely and get rid of it for good, myxopapillary ependymoma is considered a "benign" tumor. But a fragment of Morgan's tumor had been impossible to remove. Neither the initial intervention nor the healing process was straightforward for him. An infection in the wound necessitated a second surgery. And after cerebrospinal fluid began to seep down his back, a third surgery inserted a tube directing the fluid to his stomach, where his body could process it.

Medically speaking, Morgan's eventual outcome was a success. But on a personal level, it had been incredibly hard. The brutality of the operations and the radiation he had undergone for weeks, the weight loss, the initial difficulty of walking again after surgery, the withdrawal symptoms when he stopped taking the Oxycontin that had helped him through the pain. And on top of it all, the misery of having a girlfriend disappear from his life without explanation when he got sick. His parents had even moved in with him for a while to help him recover.

All this had happened a year earlier, but I wouldn't have guessed it. He had a quiet smile and took active interest in what I was saying. Nothing in the life he recounted—a full life of work, the gym, photography and convertibles, reading books and drinking Starbucks coffee at Barnes & Noble—hinted at what he had experienced so recently.

The very night of our first date, while searching for information on myxopapillary ependymoma, I realized I had a decision to make, and soon.

"Well, I don't think I'm going to die," Morgan had said. I never forgot his expression of mingled fear and strength as he said those words. If I decided to continue seeing him, I would never read any papers or research on the subject again. I didn't think it would be healthy for me.

I had three weeks of travel ahead of me to think about it and make up my mind. But I could already feel inside me, like a faint but impossible-to-miss flutter, that I was falling in love with him.

* * *

I went on my trip. As a World Bank economist, I analyze the labor market in developing countries and determine what programs, interventions and loans can offer local workers more opportunities. Even though Morgan and I had been together in person only once, for the twenty-one days that followed that meeting we exchanged emails every day. I would write him one day, he would write me back the next.

Myxopapillary ependymoma. The subject was on my mind. What should I do? My body, my desires, and my intuition were all pushing me to stay connected with Morgan. But would I risk starting a relationship with a man who had had a serious health problem that, although the doctors had given him an optimistic prognosis, I knew would be life-altering if he got sick again? Or would it be wiser to leave the relationship now, when we had seen each other only once and had made no commitment?

Arriving in my childhood town of Bahía Blanca, in southern Buenos Aires Province, to spend a few days of vacation with my family after my work assignment was a balm. I had always been very close to my mom, my dad, and my sister, even though my parents separated when I was twelve. I really needed to talk to them all. I told them everything about Morgan, our date and myxopapillary ependymoma. My parents just told me to think about it. They were afraid that I would suffer. My sister, perhaps for the first time, didn't offer an opinion. She just listened to me.

* * *

I put off the choice a little longer: at the end of September I returned to Washington, DC and to Morgan. I just wanted to see him! Though we hadn't explicitly talked about it, we were already exclusive. It's very common in online dating to date more than one person as you get to know each other. But Morgan, almost immediately after our first meeting, had removed his profiles from both Match.com and J-Date, a dating website for Jewish people. I had never thought of dating more than one person at a time, not even to test the waters, so the fact that he had stopped seeing other people to date only me struck me as a good sign.

We started to see each other very often. We went to the movies, to eat, to go cycling, to parties with friends and to play tennis. At last I had a sporting rival in my favorite activity!

As I had every year since I moved to DC, in December I planned to return to Argentina to spend the New Year's holidays with my family. I didn't have that much time to get to know Morgan better before traveling again. And I still hadn't made a final decision on whether or not I wanted to stay with him.

I was discovering that the operations had left aftereffects in Morgan. I learned these intimate details between trips to the movies and exhibitions. For example, that the surgeries had damaged so many nerves that he could not urinate without using a disposable catheter.

For example, that he had only recently resumed his work as a lawyer.

For example, that he tired quickly and was frustrated that he couldn't go camping or have the active life he had had before.

For example, that part of his shyness was due to the fact that he wasn't sure he could function sexually. One night, I confronted him about it in the car as he was dropping me off at my house.

"What's going on, Morgan. Why are you avoiding intimacy?" I asked.

"It's just that since the surgery, my testosterone levels are low. I don't know how my body's going to react to sex." His testosterone levels were low enough after his treatments that he had even stored his sperm in a sperm bank to ensure the possibility of having children in the future.

"Is there any medication or anything we can do?"

"My doctor recommended some hormones. But I don't know . . ."

"Don't worry about it. Let's just give it a try. I'm patient."

I knew Morgan didn't enjoy dating in general, because the aftermath of his surgeries meant he had to go to the bathroom all the time. But it was discouraging to find out that, despite the several dates he had been on in the last year, he hadn't had sex for long time, even before the operations. Would he want to have sex with me?

Although I reassured him during our conversation in the car, his sexual reticence and potentially atypical function bothered me, almost as much as what I had read about his illness.

Our first kiss took a while. Our "first time" was at his house. Morgan was very nervous. The stakes were high. The question of whether he was going to be able to "function," a fear for many men, was for him a real physical concern. In the end, it was much more romantic than we had thought. The way we got over that first intimacy barrier made me suspect we could overcome everything in life together. We realized that, first and foremost, what worked very well between us was something vital: communication.

* * *

"Laura, you get invited to so many parties and events. Please pick one a week you want me to attend. I'll come. But afterwards, I need time to be alone," Morgan told me one day.

That was hard for me to understand: time to be alone? But we were just beginning our love affair! And besides, I never needed to be alone. What did this need mean?

"That's me. I need my time alone, quiet, to think, I can't go out or make plans all the time," he insisted.

All my friends who met Morgan loved him. He was attentive, easy-going and charming, and held interesting conversations. One night near the end of the year I invited him to a Christmas party at the World Bank so I could introduce him to my co-workers. I saw him so relaxed, dancing and laughing, having so much fun. When the party was over, I said to him, "Shall I come sleep at your place? Or are you coming to mine?"

"No, no. I'm going back to my place," he answered.

I felt rejected. We had had a fabulous night. Why didn't he want to sleep with me? He was a tough nut to crack, this guy. Now in his forties, he had never lived with a girlfriend. Was he afraid of commitment, or was it just his reclusive personality?

I couldn't let it go. Something of the old Laura—the drama queen who fought spectacularly with all her boyfriends, who was far from the empathy and understanding that Morgan had recently awakened in me—was coming to the surface again, perhaps because of the decision I had been delaying.

After the night of that party, my phone stopped ringing. *Okay, perfect,* I thought, fuming. *We're fighting too much. He's making it easy. It looks like he decided for me. If he goes one more day without contacting me, with my month-long trip to Argentina looming, that's it.*

* * *

"Hi Laura, it's me, do you want to go to dinner tonight?"

After three days of silence, Morgan called just before I left for vacation. We had a romantic dinner at Filomena, an Italian restaurant that was one of his favorites. He apologized to me and said a lot of nice things. Among them was something I have never forgotten: that he had liked me from the moment he saw me arrive at Starbucks. That I had been on time to the date, and right on time in his life.

And as if something clicked, that night laid the solid foundation for our relationship. He understood that I needed, at times, explanations about what was happening to him: the tiredness, the restrictions that had come into his life like an unexpected visitor after the illness. I also understood that this was his personality and that his introspection was not a personal affront, that I had no reason to get angry. From then on things felt more balanced between us.

Morgan gave me peace. I liked his confidence. He knew what he wanted and, despite being a bit reserved and shy at first, he was caring and considerate. I knew I could no longer hesitate.

Somehow all of us, sick or not, live millimeters away from death, every day, every moment. It's just that no paper warns us. I was ready to put the subject of Morgan's illness out of my mind completely. I would never talk to him about the information I had found.

And so I made the best decision of my life: to stay by this man's side, whatever the future held.

CHAPTER THREE

A Family

Travel and family: both were important to both of us.

"Laura, I'm going to Las Vegas in a few days, to join my parents and my sister," he told me shortly after we started formally dating. His dad would be arriving from San Francisco; his sister, from Los Angeles. His mother would be hosting them at her home in Las Vegas.

"That's great! I'd love to come with you."

"Yeah? You want to come?"

"Of course I do!"

I knew, because he had told me, that his family wanted to meet me. After everything Morgan had been through, that he had a girlfriend was a joy for them. I got my ticket, but I wasn't on the same flight; I arrived in Las Vegas six hours before Morgan.

Tamara, his mother, picked me up at the airport. By the time Morgan arrived, I already knew dozens of family stories and had seen hundreds of pictures of him . . . even of his ex-girlfriends.

"Ah, here comes Evita Two!" his father, Nelson, said when he saw me (Morgan had had an Argentinian girlfriend before). His sister Teresa, a journalist working in television and radio—a minor celebrity, as Morgan used to joke—arrived next with the joyful news that she was pregnant. I immediately felt very comfortable with them all. Later Morgan told me they liked me as much as I liked them: "You hit the jackpot," his mother had told him. And Teresa had also given her approval, saying I was "very pretty."

Shortly after that trip, I proposed that Morgan accompany me to Argentina to meet my family. Traveling internationally, something Morgan had done a lot in his youth, had become complicated since his operations. The long hours on a plane were bad for his back. The catheter, which sometimes caused urinary infections, was difficult to use in public bathrooms. His blood sugar dropped if he did not eat every two hours, and the specific Starbucks coffee that helped him with his constipation problems was at that time not available in many other countries. Leaving the United States also meant leaving his place of comfort and safety, where he could dash to a hospital and easily communicate about any problem that might arise.

But I convinced him: we would spend two weeks visiting Buenos Aires, my hometown Bahía Blanca, and Mendoza, where my sister lived. I was delighted to show him the place where I had grown up. We visited the Club Sportiva where I had played tennis throughout my childhood and adolescence, as well as my grade school and my university. We even visited my maternal grandmother, whom Morgan found charming. They danced together and I took pictures to immortalize the moment!

"I can see why you get along well, Mari," my dad teased while we were eating together at his farm near Bahía Blanca. "You talk a lot and Morgan says yes to everything. He's very smart: I don't think he listens to half of what you say, and he doesn't challenge you!"

I started to observe Morgan and realized he *was* just like that: he always said yes, but didn't always seem to be paying attention! I'd say, "I already told you this. Don't you remember?"

On the verge of laughter, he'd reply, "I only listen to ninety-five percent of what you say!"

It became a running joke between us. It was very convenient for him, because I never knew where that famous five percent was in the conversation—at the beginning, at the end?

"Ah. It must have been in the five percent that I missed," he would say.

Despite all Morgan's doubts and fears about our trip to this faraway country, which had sounded like the Wild West to him, something in both of us relaxed in Argentina. Was it the good wine or the altitude that unwound him as the days went by? And unwound me too? Because it was on that trip, in Mendoza, that we conceived our first child.

* * *

It wasn't something we had planned. We didn't talk about the future, living together, getting married or having children. I was still renting my studio in Rosslyn and looking for an apartment to buy; he had a one-bedroom apartment nearby in Court House. But as far as sex was concerned, without talking about it or thinking about it too much, we were never careful.

With my previous boyfriends, I had taken birth control rigorously to minimize any chance of pregnancy—but not anymore. Morgan hadn't had sex with another person in a long time. Between us, the likelihood of a baby was in the air, like an unspoken agreement: we didn't plan for it, but if it came, it would be welcome. Although neither of us imagined it happening so soon!

We returned from Argentina and a month later, at the beginning of June 2009, I had to travel to a conference in Germany. When I arrived in Bonn, I realized that I had missed my period that month.

That night, after the conference was over for the day, I went out to look for an open pharmacy with Gary Fields, my PhD thesis advisor, with whom I had traveled to Germany. We were close friends. But I didn't want to take a pregnancy test without Morgan, so I called him on Skype.

It was positive!

I showed him the stick with the two pink stripes that had just changed our lives forever. I saved the picture I took on the computer of Morgan's face at that moment. I had never seen him smile so big.

*   *   *

"Let's buy a house together," Morgan said as soon as I got back from Germany.

We hadn't even left the airport. I was fresh off the plane, but still flying high—I was pregnant!—and here Morgan was, proposing that we move in together. I loved that in my absence he had been thinking about our future. That night we celebrated with salmon teriyaki at Cafe Asia, a favorite dish at a favorite spot.

Morgan was not a classic romantic. He had never said "I love you." But in small gestures like choosing that celebratory meal and, much later, surprising me with a pair of earrings that I had pointed out in a shop window, I could see and feel his love for me.

Our families were ecstatic about the pregnancy. His mother kept sending him pictures of engagement rings! It made me laugh. I was happy to have the support of his family, even though the marriage was not important to us, let alone the ring. When he asked me to move in together, I knew we were engaged. We were going to have a baby, live together, and take out a mortgage for thirty years! What bigger commitment could there be?

As my belly began, little by little, to show, we began to look for a house. At first none seemed right for us. If they were in a good neighborhood, with good schools for our future child, they were very dilapidated. If they were new houses, the prices were unaffordable. It felt like we were never going to find one.

We had the best luck around the neighborhood of "our" Starbucks. Eventually we found a house near a park in a residential neighborhood, on a small street where there were almost no cars passing by. It was a townhouse, a typical two-story brick building with a loft and a basement, a small garden in front and lots of light. It seemed like the ideal place.

I sold my old car, he sold his, we bought a Toyota Corolla. And we started to live together in our new house while we waited for the baby that was growing inside me.

* * *

For some reason, maybe because Morgan wasn't a very adaptable person, maybe because he wasn't very social—my 1500 friends on Facebook versus his 30!—or maybe because Morgan had never lived with a partner before, my new "mother-in-law" fretted that living together would drive a wedge between us.

Tamara worried that Morgan was always hot. How could we share a bed? She even had separate sheets made, European style. Her concerns seemed silly; I knew we could communicate through anything that arose.

We moved in September 2009. I had almost nothing in my studio, but Morgan had a lot of belongings for us to bring to the new house. I remember his stacks of books, the collection of cameras that he bought and sold on eBay, and especially three boxes of photographs. I looked through them all: photos of his childhood and his ex-girlfriends, photos he had taken on his travels and while playing sports. Photos of the convertible cars that he bought and sold, including a red '96 Honda del Sol that he particularly adored. And beautiful photos of his treks in nature, like in California's Yosemite National Park. It was a wonderful way to get to know him better.

Yosemite was his favorite national park, and we went back there together. I already had a big belly but we did a six-hour hike, all the way up a snow-covered mountain to Yosemite Falls. It seems crazy to me today, but I love having that wonderful picture of us—and our baby—at the top, with the snow-capped peaks all around us, touching the sky.

We enjoyed the pregnancy so much. My cousins who live in Detroit and my mom all came to spend that Christmas with us in Washington, DC, and it was all laughter and joy at the imminent arrival of our first child: a boy! Morgan and I recorded a Christmas video, me with the huge belly, both of us laughing our heads off and singing, "*Feliz Navidad, próspero año y felicidad!*" It was a special night of pure happiness.

A happiness that turned to sadness: three days before the birth of our son, my dad died.

* * *

My relationship with Morgan grew stronger day by day. The security he offered me came from his own personality, his kindness, his intelligence. The bond was solid. He gave me no reason to be jealous, and from the beginning we had told each other everything. And for me, that was especially important for family reasons: my parents had separated when I was finishing primary school because of my father Eduardo's infidelity.

Despite that, I had always had a good relationship with my dad. While I was pregnant, I wanted to spend more time together and for him to get to know Morgan better. We organized a joint trip to the Dominican Republic. Our son's photo album would start with an image of my dad kissing my belly, the sea and palm trees in the background.

We spent a few days at the beach, relaxing. I loved seeing my dad and Morgan getting along so well, even though my dad didn't speak English and Morgan didn't speak Spanish. And I was also happy that my dad saw how good our relationship was: he told me he thought it was great that Morgan was so relaxed with me.

My dad and his wife left the Dominican Republic a day before we did. We accompanied them to the airport. When we said goodbye, I had a weird feeling, which I couldn't identify at the time. I watched them leave through the gate. And that was the last time I saw my dad.

* * *

One afternoon in December, less than a month before my due date, I received a call from Argentina. It was my older half-brother, Federico, the son of the woman my dad was with before he met my mom.

Our dad had been in a car accident while driving, without a seat belt on, along Route 3 from Monte Hermoso to Bahía Blanca. He was going to see Josefina—his granddaughter, Federico's daughter—who was arriving that day from Miami, where she lived with her mother. A car had hit my father when it came suddenly out of a side road.

At that moment I did not know he had been put in a medically-induced coma and connected to an artificial respirator. My mother and my sister, who had come from Mendoza and visited him every day in the hospital, had decided not to give me much information, fearing that something might happen to me because of the advanced stage of my pregnancy. In fact, there was no longer any hope that he could be saved, but I did not know that.

I cried every night, hugging Morgan. In his arms I felt protected, and he was always aware of how I was feeling. He didn't say much, but his presence and his arms were enough for me.

While my dad was floating between life and death, serious legal and economic problems were also beginning to surface with his current wife. There were other legal issues that my sister and I had to try to agree on with Federico. It was all unwanted discussion in the middle of a coma from which my father would never wake up. And I was so far away.

* * *

Julian Eduardo Strasser was born in the afternoon of January 10, 2010 at Sibley Memorial Hospital in Washington, DC, almost a week after his due date. The day was freezing. It was a beautiful delivery, accompanied by Morgan and my mom, who traveled specially to welcome her first grandchild.

My water had broken early in the morning and the three of us rushed to Sibley. For several hours, Morgan and I plodded up and down the hospital stairs to help with dilation. The doctors finally induced my labor, as they felt there might be a risk of infection after a certain amount of time with my water broken. They gave me an epidural, so I was comfortable and really enjoyed the experience of bringing our son into the world.

I was happy and sad at the same time. In spite of my pain at not having been able to say goodbye to my dad, somehow Julian made mourning my father bearable. He showed us the incredible circle of life: some leave, others arrive, the wheel of love does not stop.

I completely forgot about work for four months. The sunlight came through the windows of my house, so new and so lovely, and everything was peaceful. Baby versions of John Lennon songs soothed us. It felt as if this little paradise was surrounded by a fluffy quilt cushioning the sadness of losing my dad, who had not even heard the news of his grandson's birth. My mom was a great help, Morgan revealed himself to be a tender and unflappable dad, and Julian was a very calm baby. During the pregnancy, I had worried a lot about something that later seemed absurd: would our baby be cute, as well as healthy? And he was. He had brown eyes with little green sparkles—he couldn't have been more beautiful.

Somehow, I felt my dad close to me at that special moment in my life. I was always talking to him in my mind. Even today, so many years later, as I write these pages, I can still feel that connection between us, a kind of virtual conversation I got used to having with him, wherever he is.

Two days after Julian was born, Morgan came over to our bed at home, where I was putting the baby to sleep.

"I love you," he said to me for the first time.

* * *

My months of maternity leave were filled by the busyness of a new mother and by a few small trips. We met up with my sister and her boyfriend in New York and improvised a baptism for Julian with holy water from St. Patrick's Cathedral.

Having proven we could do it with a baby, we kept traveling as a family when I returned to work. I convinced Morgan to come with me when I was invited to a conference in Rio de Janeiro. While I worked, Morgan took care of our son and went crazy over the scenery and the food. That first international experience encouraged me and, some time later, I traveled to Argentina by myself with the baby, where Julian got to meet his maternal great-grandmother.

We also drove all together to Detroit to see my cousins and my aunt, who had been living in the United States for years. We flew to Los Angeles to see Morgan's family, where Julian met his paternal great-grandmother. We vacationed in Miami and took a Caribbean cruise. The baby slept peacefully in his stroller while we watched shows at night. During a long walk on an island, Morgan's blood sugar dropped and we managed to get Coca Cola in a bar even though we hadn't brought any money.

Traveling together was a dream. After the operation and the difficulties of—and fears about—using the catheter and being away from his doctors, Morgan had never thought he would ever get to enjoy traveling again as he had before: without care, freely, happily. But he could.

As for daily routines, to my American friends I was, jokingly, a "bad example": Morgan never got out of bed because of the baby's cries, and I had the final say in all decisions (which we agreed upon) regarding the house and parenting.

It didn't matter to me. Morgan was more tired than usual, and anyway he was supportive, supportive, supportive and very present. His common sense seemed brilliant to me. He helped me make all kinds of decisions and gave me calm, peace and tranquility. And we divided the tasks well, in our own way.

When I had to go back to work, I also hired a nanny, Rocío. She was from Peru and Julian adored her. Today, many years later and although she no longer works with me, she is still a close friend. She was a fundamental support: she organized Julian's meals and his nap schedule. And she helped with our adult meals, the cleaning, the thousand and one details of a house revolutionized by the arrival of a baby. With that help, I could be freer to devote myself to Julian and let Morgan rest or go to the gym after work if he needed it.

Morgan loved playing and going on excursions with Julian, especially taking him to Barnes & Noble, Morgan's favorite place. Every weekend they would go to the children's section, with its books and games. Their favorite story was *The Very Hungry Caterpillar.* It was my time alone to do those things that are so difficult with a little baby: bathing quietly, waxing, talking on the phone without interruptions.

As soon as I returned to the World Bank, my boss gave me a piece of advice.

"Keep doing your romantic outings yourselves. At least once a week," he told me. "Keep going out together, because with children, the relationship changes a lot."

I thought that was wise, and so did Morgan when I told him about it. Once a week, religiously, we would go to the movies, try a new restaurant, or take a walk, while Rocío stayed with Julian. We built those extra hours into the monthly budget. It was our time: we talked about politics; about the Civil War history books Morgan was always reading; about our favorite sport, tennis; about Julian; about our friends' gossip. We went back to Filomena, reliving that important date where we had reconciled and our relationship had truly begun to grow.

We didn't talk in detail about work. I liked that he was not an economist, and that we weren't like so many of my coupled colleagues who, when they got home, were still writing papers together or discussing work-related issues. For me, coming home to or going out with Morgan was an absolute disconnection from work life, and I loved that.

Nine months after Julian's birth, we started thinking about a second child. Everything had gone so smoothly with Julian; he was such a good baby. "Why don't we try," I said, and Morgan agreed. Partly because of the aftermath of his illness, and partly because of how the dynamics of our household were, I spent more time taking care of Julian than he did, so the decision, in large part, was mine. But we were both excited and in agreement, and we decided to stop being careful.

Maybe this time it would take a while to get pregnant, as it so often does.

* * *

A month later, we were walking along Venice Beach, near Los Angeles, with Morgan's father. They had wanted to show me the house where they had lived when Morgan was a child. Julian was taking his first, tentative steps under a California sun just beginning to sink over the ocean.

In my purse I had a pregnancy test we had purchased. It was the first month since we had stopped being careful and I was overdue. I planned to take it later, maybe after the walk. But I was so nervous I couldn't wait any longer.

"I'm going to go into that bar to take the pregnancy test, Morgan. I'm not going to hold out until later," I told him.

"Ok. We'll wait for you out here," he replied.

It's another picture I treasure: Julian in Morgan's arms, the father and the mother and the son and the stick with two little pink stripes that changed our lives again. Everything was happiness.

*   *   *

Clara Fidia Strasser was born on June 28, 2011 to complete the happiness that Julian had inaugurated. She was born at Sibley, the same hospital as her brother. In just three years, Morgan and I had met, fallen in love, moved in together and conceived two children! But nothing seemed rushed to us: it had all come into our lives just in time. And when we found out our second child was a girl, we were overjoyed.

When we started talking about a name for our baby girl, I thought of Morgan's mother and sister. Tamara and Teresa are two names that have always fascinated me. And besides, they work well in both English and Spanish. However, in the Jewish religion it is not customary to name a newborn after someone who is still alive.

"I love your name," I used to say to my mother-in-law.

"No. You can't name the baby after me!" she would reply.

So my favorite choices were vetoed. During my pregnancy, my maternal grandmother passed away. In her honor, Clara's middle name is hers: Fidia, a name that apparently her parents took from Phidias, the famous sculptor from Ancient Greece. I liked that it sounded exotic.

With Clarita's arrival, we had to reorganize the household routine yet again. I couldn't take as much maternity leave this time, so Rocío would take care of Clarita. Julian, who was a year and a half old when his sister was born, finally got off the wait list and into a spot at the World Bank nursery school.

I was worried about the transition for him, though. I had read quite a bit about parenting and many books advised against making too many drastic changes with the oldest child when a second baby is born. But it was so hard to get into the Bank's nursery school! I didn't know what to do, but eventually Morgan and I decided together that Julian should start school. He had a hard time adjusting. For a month, our hearts were breaking: every time I went to pick him up, the caregiver told me that Julian had cried all day. At home, however, Julian was happy with his new baby sister. And he eventually adjusted to school, as well.

The transition was probably eased by the fact that everyone was sleeping through the night. When Julian was born, I had browsed through some parenting books at Barnes & Noble that offered methods for getting babies to sleep through the night and adapted them to my vision. It was very important to me that the baby slept well, for him and also for us, as I regained strength. I applied the same method with Clarita and it worked. In fact, both of them still sleep and rest well during the whole night, even when we travel and are on different schedules.

I resumed working and traveling for work. Morgan rarely traveled for his job: maybe a couple of times a year to New York, California or Florida. Sometimes I could even accompany him. But I was the one who spent the most time traveling, so I was always the one arranging for a babysitter and how things would work out in my absence.

Our living together was easy, despite some of Morgan's habits, such as not having regular meal times: he had to eat every two hours so his blood sugar wouldn't drop. His sweet tooth was even more voracious than mine, which meant I was trying to convince him not to consume whole pints of ice cream. He got tired easily and couldn't help around the house as much as I might have liked. In my previous relationships, there were a million things I didn't like about my partners. But with Morgan, because of his particular situation, I had no unrealistic expectations from the beginning. I always saw him as he was, and I loved him as he was.

He didn't have many domestic complaints to lodge with me either. I'm just not the most diplomatic person in the world, which sometimes showed when his parents came to visit. I loved their presence but, like any visit, it usually threw the kids' routines out of whack. I'd come home tired from work just as they finished dinner and there was their grandfather grabbing them by the feet and putting them on their stomachs, playing, laughing his head off, when we needed peace and quiet before the kids' bedtime!

Once, half jokingly and half seriously, Morgan and I created for each other little checklists titled "Things You Must Do to Make Me Happy." Each was about a hundred ideas put together in the manner of women's magazine tests, with ridiculous statements like "Agree with me," "Quit smoking" and "Don't use that voice."

I still have the one that Morgan scored for me. Out of the hundred or so sentences, he only marked four: "Calm down," "Tell me I'm sexy," "Cook" and "Cure cancer."

* * *

We made a good team. During my absences for missions with the World Bank, which can sometimes last a week or ten days in places as far away as Nepal, Uganda or Jordan, Rocío would help Morgan so he could do his job without worrying about the kids. At six o'clock in the evening, when the kids had eaten, bathed and were in pajamas, the nanny would leave and Morgan would take care of them through the night. On the weekends, he would take them to the park and Barnes & Noble. He loved playing with them.

Having been a great athlete as a kid, he dreamed of the time when he could play baseball with Julian.

One time I took Clarita with me to Argentina for a week on a work assignment. We stayed at the Four Seasons Hotel in Buenos Aires and my mom took care of her during my meeting hours. Julian stayed all that week with Morgan, who juggled work and parenting. Despite trips to the Baltimore Aquarium and the park, despite Morgan's warm and loving dedication, it was difficult for him to stay alone with Julian for a whole week.

With Clarita also came new traditions: we started renting a house for a week every August in Sea Isle City, New Jersey, three and a half hours from Washington, DC. It was almost in the middle of nowhere: the bay and picturesque villages on one side, the beach on the other. It reminded me of beaches in Argentina.

We invited family along, since the house was huge. My cousins often came from Detroit, plus my mom, of course, who always came to spend vacations with us. In the morning we'd all go down to the beach, and we'd stay until the afternoon, after the kids' nap. On the beach the kids would dig, tumble, and make sand castles. We adults loved to walk.

A favorite excursion during those beach vacations was an annual visit to the Cape May Zoo. The kids' eyes were wide as saucers at the sight of giraffes, buffalo, and giant tortoises. Sometimes, although he loved to spend time all together as a family, Morgan would take a day trip alone to Atlantic City or to the

US Open tennis tournament in New York. I understood perfectly, at this point, his need for a few moments alone.

Somehow, everything was flowing, and at the same time, everything was under control. Life was good to us, I thought, as I watched Julian and Clarita play on the shore in the sun.

CHAPTER FOUR

California Boy

In the United States, 1968 was no ordinary year. California's Summer of Love had passed and across the country the hippie dream of love and peace was slowly fading. The Vietnam War was at its height, the civil rights movement and protests on college campuses were facing police repression, Martin Luther King Jr. was assassinated in Memphis, and Bobby Kennedy, who had won the California primary in June, was fatally shot in Los Angeles. The Democratic National Convention in Chicago ended in a riot and in November Richard Nixon was elected President of the United States. *Rosemary's Baby* was released in theaters and the Beatles put out the *White Album*, two works in tune with the charged atmosphere of those times.

On September 24, 1968, the day the show *60 Minutes* debuted on television, Morgan Dov Strasser was born in Los Angeles. He was the first child of Nelson, a machine shop owner, and his wife Tamara, who worked for the Social Security Administration. The inspiration for their son's name came from David

Warner's film *Morgan*, a 1966 British comedy starring a failed artist as a bizarrely named antihero. Morgan's middle name was a tribute to his Jewish background: Dov is the name of a character in Leon Uris's novel *Exodus*, about the creation of the State of Israel.

Nelson and Tamara had met through Tamara's uncle. The couple's second child, Teresa, was born almost two years after Morgan, in June 1970. Soon the Strassers suffered their first family setback: Nelson and Tamara decided to separate when Morgan was six years old. Tamara took a job in Chicago and a judge intervened over the custody of the two siblings; Nelson was left in charge of both until Tamara returned months later to California.

When she did, the family faced a second, different separation: while Morgan stayed with his father in Venice Beach, his sister went to live with their mother nearly three hundred miles away in San Francisco. Nelson loved Morgan, but with his mother and sister far away and his father in a second relationship, Morgan lived an atypical childhood.

* * *

The Strasser family originated in Europe. Morgan's paternal great-grandfather, Bella Strasser, came in 1902 from Hungary to Ellis Island, New York, the gateway to the United States for millions of immigrants. There, officials Americanized his name to Albert, though his family continued to call him Bella. He was Jewish but not very religious. He met his wife Terez in America, though she was also Hungarian.

Bella and Terez had two sons and they made it through the hard days of the Great Depression as so many others did, through sheer hard work and perseverance. Morgan's grandfather, Edward, spoke only Yiddish and Hungarian until elementary school, but went on to win a graduate fellowship at Columbia University. He majored in finance, the same field his grandson would study many years later. A left-leaning sportsman and reader, he became president of the California employees' union and lived a long life: he died at the age of 94. Morgan was very close to his paternal grandfather and would spend many summers with his grandparents and cousins at the family home in Palo Alto.

On the maternal side, Morgan knew little of his grandparents; they died when he was still a child. Hyam, Tamara's father, was a more traditional Jew. He was very active in the Communist Party and loved Yiddish theater. Born in Russia, he was tall and strong and worked on ships during World War II. The asbestos that accumulated in his lungs from that work would degenerate into cancer years later. Mildred, Morgan's maternal grandmother, was Polish. Morgan remembered only how much he loved going to her house for kreplach dinner. Tamara was the only child of the couple, who had both had other children with their previous partners.

* * *

Morgan excelled at sports as a child. Atypically for a boy raised between Santa Monica and Venice

Beach, he didn't surf, but he did have a special talent for tennis—at the age of nine he was beating adults—for padel (another raquet sport) and above all for baseball. A leftie, he was a star bat in Little League starting at age seven. Suddenly at age twelve, though, he couldn't hit the ball anymore. Nelson took him to the ophthalmologist; it seemed like his vision had diminished considerably. But no: according to the specialist, his vision was still perfect. It's a mystery why he could not continue playing baseball, a sport in which he had been so talented. His vision seemed to deteriorate in that game but not in tennis. Later, he would need to wear glasses throughout his life.

While he was passionate about sports—in photos from his teenage years he is always biking, rock climbing, camping, playing ping pong, and diving in San Francisco to catch abalone, which he loved—he left much to be desired in academics. Nelson had remarried, to a psychologist, and they had moved to Santa Rosa with Morgan and their three children, one of whom was schizophrenic. Morgan lived in a small room in the garage. He was still far from his own mother and sister, and his father's new wife was not particularly loving to him. The challenging dynamics of his home life began to show as rebelliousness at school. He was kicked out again and again because of his behavior. He got bad grades; academics didn't seem to interest him.

His last semester at Santa Rosa Junior High was disastrous. He and two friends brought a lemon shark from Santa Monica and threw it into a motel pool. Because of this and other shenanigans, he had to sit for an interview with a school psychologist. The first thing the psychologist said to Nelson after the interview was, "This kid is loaded."

Nelson thought the worst: that Morgan was on drugs. But the psychologist was referring to Morgan's high IQ. His family realized his behavior might have been stemming partly from boredom at school. They finally decided he could move to be with his mother and sister in San Francisco. He started therapy and his personality changed remarkably. He went from being a "little dictator," who bossed around all his teammates in baseball and smoked marijuana at the age of twelve, to being a quiet and studious boy, never in a bad mood.

In eighth grade at Drew College Prep, a school for seventh through twelfth grade that offered many Advanced Placement classes, Morgan discovered his passion for history. He was stimulated at school by engaging teachers and tough assignments. And he pulled together the grades to graduate with honors and go to the University of Berkeley.

Morgan also met his life-long best friend, Phil, at Drew. A ping pong table and Morgan's extraordinary talent for the game brought them together.

* * *

Morgan's first idea was to study medicine at Berkeley. At one point, he took a chemistry class that combined two semesters into one and required a score of 700 on the math section of the SAT, a national standardized test necessary to begin a college career. Morgan had a 680. The professor wanted to include him anyway, in a very competitive class. Despite Morgan's good grades and the fact that he had the temperament and intellect for a career in medicine, it was an arduous path, and he decided to leave medicine in favor of finance.

After a year of living on campus, Morgan moved into an apartment with Phil and Phil's siblings. In the summers, he traveled: backpacking Europe, an internship in Hong Kong, exploring Thailand, even a trip to Japan after college. While he was pursuing a finance degree at Berkeley, his sister Teresa was studying journalism on the East Coast at New York University. She would go on to become a well-known, Emmy Award-winning radio and television host.

At Berkeley, Morgan met Michelle, his first serious girlfriend. But it didn't last long beyond college. Morgan decided to pursue a career in law and moved from Berkeley to Santa Clara to do his J.D. at the local law school. Phil also moved there and they continued to share their daily life in an apartment five minutes from campus. When Morgan and I first met, I always joked that what he had done was not really a doctorate: there are the medical doctors, who are the real doctors; then the economics PhDs, like me; and then there are the *Juris Doctor* cheaters like Morgan, who only need to do two years of post-college study.

Morgan's forte had always been mathematics, like his mother, who had had excellent grades during her years at UCLA. Morgan turned that skill into a specialization in estate tax law. He ended up working for the federal government managing property taxes as applied to inheritances on international estates. It was a very secretive job: Morgan did not talk about it and I once learned only by chance that he had handled the estate tax for the Australian actor Heath Ledger, who had lived and died in the United States.

Morgan liked that his job was quiet. When he was eventually offered a managerial position, he declined. He preferred data analysis, a more technical task, to managing people, even if the latter meant a promotion. But he was generous with his knowledge: he never turned away a finance question from a colleague, and more than once he helped his father with work problems or contractual issues.

Morgan's most serious relationship before we met was with a second Michelle. Their relationship always made me jealous, maybe because of the dozens of photos of her that Morgan had kept, maybe because of how in love Morgan had been, maybe because she had left him and became a kind of obsession for him for a while.

From Santa Clara Morgan went to Cincinnati, Ohio, where he lived for four years. And from Cincinnati he went to Washington, DC—where both Phil and Mike, his other best friend from Berkeley, were already living—in 2005, the same year I arrived in that city. In between, starting in the late 1990s, his back pains began.

* * *

Glad to be back in proximity to his friends, Morgan would watch with them over and over again classic comedies like *The Big Lebowski* and *The Tao of Steve*. But unlike Cincinnati, DC also offered plenty to do outside the house. Morgan loved visiting museums, riding around in a convertible, and eating bagels and drinking coffee while browsing the latest books in the history and politics section at Barnes & Noble. From DC it was easy for him to travel to New York to watch the US Open. He even took private flying lessons.

When his mother Tamara—as much of a gourmet as Morgan—visited him, they loved to have special dinners together. They didn't mind, for example, driving an hour and a half to try a restaurant famous for its menu, such as The Inn at Little Washington. Morgan and his father Nelson had always shared a love of nature and sports. Once Morgan settled in Washington, DC, on Nelson's visits they loved to ride bikes along the Potomac River to Alexandria or Mount Vernon together, or go for a drive to historic sites, such as Thomas Jefferson's home in Monticello. Over the years, Morgan had kept his keen interest in history, whether it was the Civil War or the Cuban Missile Crisis in the 1960s. His father matched those interests with enthusiasm. They loved spending time together.

Although deep down he would always miss California a little, in Washington, DC, Morgan would find a certain direction for his life. Living in the same city without knowing each other, I was on the same quest.

CHAPTER FIVE

From South to North

On March 29, 1975, while Morgan was facing the separation of his parents in California, I was born more than six thousand miles away in Bahía Blanca, a prosperous port city on the Argentine Sea, south of the province of Buenos Aires, on the border with Patagonia.

Like Morgan, I came into the world at a turbulent time. Argentina was being governed by Isabel Martínez de Perón, who ascended from the vice presidency to the presidency after the death of her husband, President Juan Domingo Perón, in July 1974. Between murders by the paramilitary organization Triple A, guerrilla coups, and severe economic devaluation, the country was facing one of the most violent years in its history. A year after my birth, the country would enter its darkest period: a military dictatorship would rule until 1983.

However, even in turbulent times people enjoy, behind closed doors, some of the happiest events of private life, and for my parents the birth of their first daughter on that hot March 29th was one of them.

* * *

My whole family had been settled in Bahía Blanca for two generations. One of my maternal great-grandfathers was Italian and in Bahía Blanca he built a car dealership, Corbatta Hermanos, which became very well known. My other maternal great-grandfather came from Spain. My maternal grandparents, Ricardo Corbatta, whom we called "Yeyi," and Fidia Santos, whom we called "Bele," were born in Bahía Blanca. Yeyi—studying to become an accountant—and Bele—a great cook, elegant and energetic—got married when she was nineteen years old. They lived in the province of Chaco for a while but returned to Bahía Blanca when my mother, Graciela, was born. They lived together for almost sixty years, until my grandfather's death, and I was able to enjoy their company as I grew up.

My paternal grandfather, Antonio Sánchez, came to Bahía Blanca from Spain when he was eight years old. Antonio, who was an accountant and a representative of a small soccer club in the city, married my grandmother María Elena Puerta Durcudoy, who was born in Puán. They had three children. Their life together was difficult until Antonio opened a shop selling agricultural spare parts, a business that his children would inherit. He died of a heart attack when my father, Eduardo, was twenty years old.

I did not get to know Antonio, but I do remember my grandmother, a loving and very religious woman. She died when I was twelve years old. One Friday in 1986, she fell off the balcony of her house. Or she jumped off the balcony. It was never clear. My dad was on a trip and learned of her death when he returned. It was a hard blow for him.

* * *

Twelve years older than my mom, my dad fell in love with her while they were both working at the National University of the South. In addition to managing several farms on the outskirts of the city and expanding the agricultural parts and diesel engine business he had inherited from his father, my dad was a professor of financial administration in the accounting program. Graciela was an assistant in his class.

The relationship did not start right away. When they met, my father was in another relationship and had a son, Federico, and my mother was about to marry a boyfriend, whom she ended up leaving. Once they were together, social pressures made the relationship a challenge. In the seventies, in a city with the soul and gossip of a small town, where everybody knows everybody, a recently separated man and a young girl were the perfect target for disapproving looks.

My parents got married on September 5, 1974. It was the first marriage for both of them. My dad's first partner was divorced and, under Argentina's laws at the time, she and my dad had not been able to get married. And it would also be the only marriage for both my dad and my mom: although they separated when I finished primary school, they were never legally divorced. It took me years to connect dates and realize that my mom was pregnant with me when they got married. That version of the script is common now but in those years was always kept secret.

A year and a half after my birth, the family was completed with the arrival of my sister, Maria Virginia, nicknamed Vir. For whatever strange reasons exist in the internal nebula of each family, Vir and I would only start having contact with our half-brother Federico when we were teenagers. Today the three of us adore each other.

* * *

My childhood was spent in downtown Bahía Blanca. My father split his time between the countryside and the university. My mother also worked part-time at the university and was very devoted to Vir and me. We spent our summers in a little apartment in front of the sea on Monte Hermoso beach. Over time, summers on that beautiful beach where the sun sets over the sea at dusk became one of our most valued family traditions. Even today, it is the most anticipated time of the year for my own children.

Vir and I were always great companions and friends. We went together to primary school N°4, three blocks away from our house, and we spent our weekends at Club Sportiva, one of the most respected clubs in town, playing tennis or swimming in the pool in the summer.

Tennis is a passion we inherited from our mother. In the early eighties, with tennis player Guillermo Vilas becoming a popular idol, the sport was also in fashion. Since my mother had only been allowed to play tennis at home when she was a teenager, she wanted us to be able to enjoy it in public from an early age. And boy, did we enjoy it.

I quickly started to love tournaments, unlike Vir who, although she was and still is a great player—probably better than me—was very nervous when facing a competition. I played in local, regional and, after age seventeen, national tournaments. I also participated in first category competitions, separate high-level tournaments without age restrictions. I took it very seriously. I trained two or three days a week; tennis drills were great, though I was always trying to find an excuse to get out of the extra hour of just running. I spent many weekends traveling for tournaments. I had no ambitions to be number one but I enjoyed and was stimulated by the competition.

As much as I enjoyed competing on the tennis circuit, my attitude at school was less bold. I was shy, and in primary school I spent hours alone writing, reading, drawing, and studying languages. While Vir said she wanted to be a veterinarian, I said I was going to be a writer, like my aunts. Both my mom's sister, Jorgelina Corbatta, who today lives in Detroit and is a renowned academic, and my dad's brother's wife, Titi, were writers. Titi gave me notebooks and encouraged me to write.

I loved theater. I made up little plays with lots of dialogue and participated in theater workshops in school. I also wrote short stories. The local newspaper, *La Nueva Provincia*, had a children's supplement on Sundays, called *Totópolos*. They published some of my stories when I was seven or eight years old. My mother still has them. One of them seems significant to me, in light of the decisions I have made in my life. It is about two girls who arrive at a cave and, although they are afraid, decide to go in rather than return to the safety of home.

I WRITE, YOU WRITE... THE TALE OF THE CAVE

They were two good friends named Lucía and Lucrecia. They always met at school or at games.

One day they came to a cave and did not know what to do, they were scared to death, whether to enter the cave or go home, so they decided to enter the cave.

They thought it was full of candy (they loved candy), so they entered the cave, where they did not find candy but a giant who said to them with a voice like thunder:

"Who came into my cave?"

"Lucía and Lucrecia."

"Let's go home," said one of them, "I'm afraid."

"Yes, yes, let's go home."

The giant prepared to close the cave door and the friends hurried out of the cave.

When they got home, they told their mother everything and she told them never to get into mischief again, and they obeyed her.

And by golly, this story is over.

María Laura Sánchez Puerta
Bahía Blanca

My shyness, my seeking refuge in writing and languages, likely came in part from my body. I was self-conscious about my hair, a lion's mane with no shape at a time when the ideal of beauty demanded straight and long hair. And I have a birthmark: a red tide that extends from my hand along my right arm, chest and shoulder blade. I would be lying if I said I had totally overcome my self-consciousness about it, even now.

But, like so many vulnerable feelings, it was worse in childhood and adolescence. I still remember some incidents as if they were today. Once, during one of the national tennis tournaments, the girl I was going to play against noticed my birthmark. I was wearing a sleeveless T-shirt and it was clearly visible. I explained to her what it was.

"And how do you do it on the beach?" she asked me.

Her question kept rattling around in my head. *What do I do on the beach? I put on my bikini. And that's it,* I repeated mentally while we played. Channeling my anger in every serve, in every backhand, I roundly beat her. I was delighted to have won even one match at that level of competition.

Boys were especially cruel about other people's peculiarities. The popular television show *Adderly* featured a detective who wore a black glove, and boys used it as an excuse to tease me about my hand.

I had a few friends—I'm still friends with them, in fact—but I didn't connect with the popular kids in class, who could sing all the trendy songs on the radio. I didn't even know what music was playing. And I only seemed to develop impossible crushes on boys I never spoke to or who were the coolest in tennis and never looked at me. That shyness would change during secondary school. As would so many other things.

* * *

Just before I started my first year of secondary school—which in Argentina happens around age thirteen— my mom discovered my dad's infidelity. They tried a reconciliation; when it didn't work, they decided to separate. I don't remember it particularly affecting Vir and me. It hurt us more to see Mom so sad. In the middle of lunch, she would burst into tears and run to her room.

She tried to rebuild her life. She started to grow a lot in her job and would eventually become the director of the School of Commerce at the National University of the South. She never, in spite of her pain, spoke badly of my father. In fact, since they were both professors, she continued working with him for many years. In spite of their separation, they were able to treat each other cordially. He moved into an apartment and Vir and I saw him a lot; we'd have lunch during the week or go to the countryside together on weekends.

The separation never directly damaged my relationship with my dad, but it did leave a mark. I have never stopped puzzling over why men cheat. To this day I devour books or series like *Mad Men* to try to understand unfaithful men. And, later in my life, I always chose boyfriends who were the opposite of a Don Juan.

But back when the separation was a recently opened wound, I wasn't thinking about boyfriends. I was preparing myself through private classes to take the very competitive entrance exam to the Basic Cycle of the School of Commerce—the same institution where my mother would later become director. I came in second out of two thousand applicants.

*　*　*

When I started secondary school there, I was still the same withdrawn girl who in primary school was made fun of as the one with the lion's hair, the nerd who studied a lot. The School of Commerce was very demanding; while most secondary schools in Argentina are five-year programs, ours was six years. I was in the best level, since they were ordered by proficiency in English, and mine was excellent. But I felt very insecure both socially and about my body. Going out shopping was torture and sometimes I preferred not to go to big parties like quinceañeras if it meant I had to get something new to wear.

Around age fifteen, I started to write in a diary every night about the events of the day: a tennis tournament in General Suarez where I won and the prize was a pair of sneakers and a cup, the day I took my friend Mariel to my dad's field and we went horseback riding with my dog Trompita. I also pondered more philosophical questions: What did I want to do with my life?

Around the same time, although I continued to be a good student, I finally stopped demanding quite so much of myself at school. This gave me some space to finally begin making friends. Nicolas was the first one, one of the coolest kids in my school division. I used to help him study. Becoming friends with him gave me fresh and powerful confidence: I could be friends with these guys! They were not so different from me! Nicolas was the key that unlocked my social side.

* * *

Although she only spent three years in Bahía Blanca, my friend Mariel profoundly shaped who I was and planted the seed of a dream that would come true. The daughter of a military man stationed at the base in Bahía Blanca, she entered my primary school in sixth grade. We became close friends. She came from Washington, DC; that she had lived in another country seemed both exotic and exciting. Traveling and seeing the world became one of my strongest desires. I had no idea how I could achieve it.

My first chance came in my fifth year of secondary school. Another friend's mother represented the Youth for Understanding (YFU) organization and asked me if I was interested in doing a student exchange program in the United States. Of course I was interested! I ran to propose it to my parents and they were so enthusiastic that they agreed to finance the trip. I would live in a family home for six months and study in English *if* I could pass the entrance exam.

No one told me how to prepare. It turned out to be a general test on US culture and history. How many stars are on the American flag? Who were the most important presidents? I took the test at the YFU representative's house, and she helped me with the answers. I passed the test. I was in: I would go to high school in the United States!

* * *

People from Buenos Aires who applied to YFU went to places like Boston or San Francisco. I, who came from Bahía Blanca, was sent to a town they considered equivalent to my hometown: Elwood, a wasteland of ten thousand inhabitants in middle-of-nowhere Indiana. I arrived in the dead of winter at a farm far from town, where I was greeted by a charming older couple. Over the years they had hosted about thirty exchange students, some while their children—now married and themselves with children—were going to high school in Elwood.

It was a shock. I took in the snow, the farm, how far it was to drive to town by myself, and how far, far away I was from my family. That first day, I was overcome with regret.

Communication with my family was once a week, by letter. My hosts drove me to and from school, and I didn't have many activities to concentrate on besides academics. I did become friends with other exchange students, especially Jose, a Dutch girl I still keep in touch with and whom I frequently visit when I stop in Amsterdam on business trips.

Since I didn't have much distraction, I focused on two things at hand. One was tennis, which I practiced every day. I quickly started winning tournaments, even reaching the state finals in Indianapolis, the capital of Indiana. The other was food, always readily and plentifully available. Cake with ice cream for dessert every day, chocolate milk and pizza for lunch . . . despite my training schedule I put on fifteen pounds in those six months.

Toward the end of the exchange I was offered a scholarship to a college in Indiana, where I could play tennis and study at the same time. But I still didn't know what career I wanted to pursue, and besides, I missed my family terribly. I didn't even consider it: it was time to go home.

* * *

I returned to Argentina in June, at the American summer break but in the middle of the Argentinian school year. My original idea had been to fold back in with my old classmates and finish my sixth year at the School of Commerce, but I had missed too much of their specific, demanding curriculum to start at that point in the year. Besides, with the months in the United States added onto the five of my school's six years I had done before I left, I had already completed a normal secondary school cycle. I received my diploma.

My dad suggested I take advantage of it and start college right away. But in Argentina you choose a set course of study right at the start, and I had no idea what career path to follow. I liked History. My dad suggested Economics instead. He told me within Economics I'd study history, law, and other subjects that were a good base for further study, and that a degree in Economics would let me do whatever I wanted later on.

I enrolled at first in History and Economics at the National University of the South and eventually settled on just Economics, as my dad had suggested. I didn't even consider the possibility of going to college in Buenos Aires; during the exchange I had missed my home so much and this program was a very good one, anyway.

That first year was hard, a déjà vu of my shyness as a girl. All the students already knew each other because they had started their studies a semester before and it was difficult to fit in. In each class, I took exhaustive notes on what the professors explained and wrote down all my questions. At the end of class, when everyone else wanted to leave as quickly as possible, I would approach the professor to try and get answers. My classmates, once again, saw me as a nerd.

My shyness and physical self-consciousness returned, amplified by the pounds I had gained during my stay in the United States. However, I soon began to feel and look better. One rare night—I have always liked daytime activities more than nightlife—I went dancing at a bowling alley. And there I met Diego, my first love and my boyfriend on and off for the next seven years.

* * *

I liked him at first sight, when he walked up to me and asked, "Do you want to dance?" An engineering student at the same university as me, Diego was tall, skinny, brown-haired, and sporty looking. I thought he was beautiful. We got together immediately.

Diego and his family were struggling. His sister was disabled, the family had little income, and Diego had a course of study that demanded too much from him considering he also had to work. I had demands for him that I later understood were too much, too, like that he should be more sociable or that we should go out more. In a moment of great pressure, he decided to break off our relationship. It was a surprise to me.

My dad was my confidant. Whenever I needed him, I could find him in the afternoons playing basketball at Club Argentino. I went to look for him the day Diego wanted to break up, and started crying when I saw him. It was my first great sorrow of love. And he knew how to console me; I'll never forget that bear hug he gave me. Three days later, Diego wanted to see me. We made up.

*   *   *

During my college years, I was a teaching assistant at the university in a couple of subjects and won several merit scholarships, all of which cemented my academic confidence. In my fourth year, I began to pay attention to the ads posted on the university bulletin boards announcing internships. And so it was that one summer I went to the city of Campana, in the north of the province of Buenos Aires, for an internship with the Techint company. It was another world: there were interns from other countries and I felt independent, happy and adventurous. I felt that I no longer wanted to be a girlfriend, and I broke off my relationship with some ridiculous excuse.

Half a lifetime later, I can understand that twenty-two-year-old Laura was eager to take on the world and dazzled by the possibility of an interesting job, a very good salary, colleagues from places so different from Bahía Blanca . . . But every fairy tale has its end and, when I returned home after that summer, I realized I was coming back to reality. And the reality was that I still wanted to be with Diego.

*   *   *

Diego took me back as I was in the final stretch of my studies. I graduated with a degree in Economics and my thesis director, Silvia London, helped me win a research grant that would enable me to get a PhD. I wasn't particularly interested in academic life, but I knew I needed to keep moving forward while I thought about how my life would continue. I hoped during the PhD new options would appear . . . and they did.

A well-connected professor who had studied in the United States, Fernando Thome, noticed my good GPA and my ability to study. He insisted that I apply for the Fulbright scholarship to get a doctorate in the United States. The misery of my exchange studies in desolate Indiana was seven years behind me. And after my positive experience at Techint, I was more amenable to the idea of leaving Argentina for a challenge that, I was sure, could open the door to my future career.

The scholarship funded the PhD in Economics but, if I managed to do well in my first year, I would be guaranteed a master's degree and wouldn't have to continue for four more years for my PhD if I didn't want to. I went in expecting to get my master's degree and then to return home.

I traveled to Buenos Aires to take the Fulbright exams. I applied to five American universities. Of all of them, my favorite was Cornell, in Ithaca, New York. But I didn't tell Diego about it, thinking maybe I wouldn't even get the scholarship. But I did. My life was changing again.

"What? Are you thinking of leaving?"

I can't forget Diego's disconsolate face. I didn't know how to explain to him how much I was interested in this. It was unlikely that he could tear himself away from his computer engineering job, his studies, and his complicated family situation to come with me. For a while he thought maybe he could apply for some scholarship and we could go together. But nothing came of it for Diego, and I left in August 2000. I would be back in six months for the holidays, and we planned to figure out then how to continue our story together. I planned never to spend more than a year away, and we thought we could be in a long-distance relationship.

I thought that way because I didn't imagine what I would find in Ithaca. What I found was a superb university, so many possibilities within my reach, sudden access to international organizations that sent people with my skills on trips all over the world . . . Bahía Blanca, and all that it implied, seemed smaller and smaller.

*   *   *

I arrived in Ithaca in the middle of the summer, at night, to a house on the outskirts of campus that I was to share with a French girl, a Chinese girl and an American girl. Among my classmates there was only one other Argentinean, but I shared courses with Indians, Mexicans, Kenyans and Germans.

The relationship with Diego became more and more deflated. A German boy began to court me. I was interested in him and we became close friends, but the infidelity issue weighed on me and I made sure nothing happened between us. But when I returned to Bahía Blanca for the holidays at the end of my first semester at Cornell, Diego and I ended our seven-year relationship for good. I had already decided that I wanted to stay in the US to apply for a three-month internship at the World Bank. Our paths had simply diverged too much.

I adapted very well to the demanding university life. I treasured the American values of diversity and flexibility, the acceptance of being who you are and the transparency of earning things with your own effort. No longer under the sway of the small-town atmosphere that made me feel different and judged, I gained a lot of confidence. My sister Vir did a PhD in Biology at the University of Maryland and a post-doctorate in Indiana but returned to Argentina as soon as she was done. Unlike her, in the United States I now felt happy and at home.

* * *

That first year I didn't get the World Bank internship, but I had already set that kind of job as a long-term goal. Academia didn't appeal to me. I didn't see myself as a professor or a university researcher, nor being alone in an office day in and day out. Working in an international organization, on the other hand, seemed ideal for me.

Thanks to Ramya, one of the smartest students in my class, with whom I used to study, I passed the very difficult exams of that first year of my PhD. Then I met my advisor, Gary Fields, who was indispensable in helping me choose research directions. He himself worked a lot with the World Bank. I gave him tennis lessons, so I had the advantage of spending extra time with him and being able to talk through my doubts and questions with him. We still exchange messages on birthdays and holidays, and meet at conferences. "I'm so proud of you," he often comments when I post on social media about my work.

Those early days at Cornell seemed crazy to many because everyone barely lifted their heads out of their books. Though I had as many insecurities as any freshman, I never doubted my ability to enjoy life even in difficult times. When I wasn't studying, I was traveling. Some travel was for economics conferences, but much was for fun. I visited my cousin Pepe Sanchez, who had been an NCAA basketball star at Temple University and was drafted into the NBA my first semester in the States. He was the first Argentinian to play in the league. I also traveled often to Greek Peak, a nearby ski resort that had cheap passes for students. And in the middle of the academic year, New York's winter but Argentina's summer, I always went to Bahía Blanca to visit my family.

* * *

I got the research internship at the World Bank at the end of the second year of my PhD. I was part of a group that studied poverty in Latin America. Since everything at the university is more theoretical than practical, everything I learned at the World Bank was very useful for me when writing my thesis. An Argentinian researcher there, Guillermo Cruces, even provided me with data from the permanent household survey in Argentina that became the basis of my dissertation.

By that time, I had already had my first American boyfriend, Finn. The relationship had lasted a year but made me realize that I did not want to have a boyfriend who did the same work as me; Finn was very insecure and talked all day long about economics and PhD issues. After him, I met Carlos, an Argentinian who was doing a graduate degree at Cornell but soon moved to Colorado. I didn't mind the distance. I was so happy with our relationship that I went to visit him often. On one of those trips, after we had been dating for six months, Carlos gave me a surprise.

"Are you crazy? You make me come all the way out here and then break up with me?" I said. "Please get me the ticket to go back to Ithaca right away. I want to leave."

That same day I went back to school and never thought about him again. I focused on the hardest thing: the path to my doctoral dissertation. My thesis was on labor mobility in Argentina from 1993 to 2003, a subject that would later interest the World Bank since it was related to issues they work on there. But writing it was excruciating: after classes, study and friendships, you face the blank paper and are alone in front of your ideas and theories. I thought many times I would not make it. But at last, I pulled the threads together, and I got my doctorate in 2005. I already knew that I did not want to return to Argentina. I had discovered my dream job.

* * *

Before that, there was Jean Carlos. Or "Yan," as I called him. He was a Colombian guy who was doing a PhD in Mathematics and whom I met in my last year at Cornell. We knew the same people and soon became close friends. When he finished his PhD, I was in the final stretch of my dissertation. He went to Ohio to work as a professor but called me every day. I didn't think anything could happen between us because I wasn't that attracted to him physically, but he was very intelligent and charming and we had a lot of interests in common.

Yan ended up making me fall in love over the phone. He came to visit me when I graduated and, though I've never been sure *exactly* how it happened, we ended up spending the night together. Thus began a long-distance relationship that lasted three years: first between Washington, DC, and Ohio, then between Washington, DC, and Colombia. Because after I graduated, my dream job became a reality: in August 2005 I moved to the capital of the United States to fulfill a two-year contract at the World Bank.

I was very excited to work in research as a labor economics consultant with a mission to eradicate poverty. I got to work in developing countries, to travel and to collaborate with very interesting people from around the world. I was assigned to work in the Europe and Central Asia region, and I started to travel to Serbia, Turkey and Germany for conferences and reports on the labor market.

I hoped to make the World Bank placement permanent, but Yan insisted that I look for a job in Bogotá, Colombia, so that I could be with him. A little to please him, a little to see if I was closing myself off to an interesting option, I applied to one of the most important universities in Bogotá. They offered me an academic job . . . at the same time the World Bank offered me a permanent position in a central unit in Washington, DC, analyzing labor market data and interventions to solve global unemployment.

It was a no-brainer. Yan was determined to stay in Colombia; there was no chance that he would move to where I had work projects. He said he wanted to marry me and for us to live in Colombia, and that I was very selfish for not wanting to leave my job for him. Yan did not want to live in the United States and I felt that, despite being very bohemian and intellectual, he was not flexible at all. I decided to end the relationship.

*   *   *

My first year working at the World Bank was tough. I had gone from the familiar world of the university to a completely different environment. And

I didn't have a welcoming home to come back to at the end of each day. My roommate, whom I had found through the Internet, made my life impossible. She wanted to control me, she always told me that it was her house rather than ours, she didn't like me to be sociable and bring friends over, she didn't like Yan visiting me, and she made me look bad when my mom came from Argentina to spend a few days with me.

I had been staying late at the office many nights and feeling very unproductive. One day my director passed by my office, backtracked to watch me, and said, "Laura. Stop eating ice cream." I was cradling a pint in my lap, soothing my frustration with food. His words were a wake-up call.

Little by little, I realized my aspirations were being fulfilled. The Bank was a motivating place, teeming with engaging people. My work was a combination of analysis, travel in contact with the people of the country the Bank seeks to help, and connection with the governments that draw on its analysis to improve their economic and social policies. Above all, I had the satisfaction of seeing practical results from my work.

It was a stimulating job based in a city I liked very much, with the possibility of getting to know the world. I had left my oppressive housing situation the moment the lease was up. All I needed now was to meet someone with whom I could really share my life. And it was then—just in time—that Morgan, the guy from Match.com, came into my life.

CHAPTER SIX

The Word I Cannot Pronounce

August 2013. We were staying for the weekend in cabins in the Shenandoah Mountains, three hours from home. I had won the trip in a store raffle and we invited my mom, who was now babysitting the kids. The suitcases were already loaded in the car; we were heading back to DC that afternoon. Before we did, I got to relish one of my greatest pleasures, rare since we became parents: challenging Morgan, my best opponent, to a tennis match.

The place was beautiful and had some pretty good cement courts. We started with a warm-up rally. Morgan was running, taking it very seriously. So was I. This time I was sure I'd beat him, a glorious finishing touch to a lovely summer weekend.

* * *

"Lau, let's stop for a while," Morgan told me after a setback.

"What's the matter?"

"My back hurts. A lot. Did I strain it too much getting the suitcases into the car?"

That afternoon Morgan drove us home, though the pain wouldn't let up.

"Let's go see Dr. Gokaslan," I suggested.

At that point, almost six years after the myxopapillary ependymoma operation, Morgan was seeing his doctor once a year for an MRI checkup. I would have been more at ease—much more—if the check-ups were every six months. I knew that, in his first operation, they had not been able to remove all the tumor from his spine without risking his life. And I sometimes worried knowing that this type of tumor can begin to metastasize to the brain, though that's not too common in adults.

The last thing Morgan wanted was to be in a closed device, sitting still for more than an hour. Every year, when the blessed checkup came, he would take a tranquilizer before the MRI. But we made an appointment with Dr. Gokaslan at Johns Hopkins Hospital in Baltimore, where he had operated on Morgan in 2007, and a couple of weeks later I accompanied him to the post-MRI consultation.

The pain still wouldn't let up. The diagnosis was clear: there was a microincision in the titanium prosthesis they had used to replace part of Morgan's vertebra after removing the tumor. That is to say, there were two tiny titanium "rods" in his back, one of which had broken. It meant his back had to be operated on yet again.

Given the constant microfriction inside the body, the break wasn't a surprise to Dr. Gokaslan. But it was a surprise to us. I felt indignation and fear rising like a fever. If this had always been a possibility, why wasn't Morgan warned? He played tennis, carried suitcases. Should he not have exerted himself so much? Both Morgan and I knew that the operation, though simple, could turn into a cascade of interventions. Every procedure Morgan had undergone in the past was followed by infection and fever and all sorts of cumbersome problems.

"How can this be?" I wondered aloud.

"Laura, in general, the prostheses are very resilient," Dr. Gokaslan reassured me. "And what we as doctors want is for Morgan to have a good quality of life. If we operate on him for a tumor, but then he can't live a normal life, it's like he's still sick."

I calmed down a little bit. We both did. Dr. Gokaslan was the only one who knew the case inside and out and could read the MRI with minimal chance of error; intricate scar tissue showed up in the imaging and could confuse the diagnosis. If he said it was necessary to operate, then it had to be done.

* * *

In the midst of the additional tests that Dr. Gokaslan ordered, the pain began to subside. September passed, October arrived. At that month's consultation, it was decided that Morgan would have surgery at Johns Hopkins Hospital on November 7. I had a work trip to Jordan in early November; the operation would be on my return. Nelson, Morgan's father, would come be with Morgan and help us with the kids as well. He could stay at the hospital in Baltimore with Morgan while I went back to DC to spend the night with Julian and Clarita. For my work there was no major inconvenience: the job was always very flexible, I had consultants to help me, and I could continue working from the hospital.

Julian and Clarita were very young and had to continue with life as normally as possible. "Dad's back is hurt," we told them, "and he is going to stay a few days at the doctor's so he can heal." We always told them everything. I don't know how much they understood rationally, but they knew something was wrong. One day Julian put a little glass ball in his nose—a totally atypical behavior. I called his pediatrician in desperation and she reassured me that surely the little ball had passed to his stomach. Some time later, Clarita imitated him. I didn't know what to do, my children were rebelling! It was clear that they were expressing their distress in their own way.

* * *

After five hours of surgery to replace the titanium rods and two days in the hospital, Morgan came home. Of course, we had to take special care as in any post-operative period. There were two small tubes draining fluid from his back that we had to empty and clean. Other than that, he was allowed to go back to his normal life, including work. I tried to hide my panic. What if the tubes came out? Or what if he crushed them when he lay down and the wound came open?

Even as he tried to regain normalcy, the domino of interventions we feared happened. He started running a fever, something to monitor closely. The antibiotics made him nauseous. Within a week of the operation, the nausea was so bad that we had to take him to the emergency room. And two weeks later, out of the blue, his fever was so high that we had to go directly to Johns Hopkins. Morgan was admitted. The doctors did a lumbar puncture, or spinal tap, to assess Morgan. It was decided that the best thing to do was to put him on an IV to pass antibiotics directly into his blood. Tamara, his mom, arrived to help us with the logistics. I started driving back and forth from Washington, DC to Baltimore every day on a triangular circuit between our home, the hospital and my job at the World Bank.

It was already December when he returned home, recovered. We had missed Thanksgiving, so we made a feast: Tamara cooked turkey and all the typical Thanksgiving dishes. We invited some friends over. Morgan went back to work yet again, and I started planning my annual trip to Argentina for the holidays. Everything was slowly getting back to normal, but I asked Tamara to please stay with Morgan until I returned.

*   *   *

The beaches of Monte Hermoso, very close to Bahía Blanca, have always been my refuge, and that of my family. Every December or January I traveled there from the United States with the kids—sometimes Morgan would join us. My sister Vir came from Mendoza with her husband and her daughters to spend some time with my mom in the little apartment we have in front of the beach. It is the highlight of our year.

I knew that, after all the stress we had been through, the best thing for the kids and for me, the most restorative thing, would be this vacation. Morgan was very insistent that we travel. He was fine, he felt fine, he was going to be well taken care of by his mother. I, however, was reluctant to leave. Communication wasn't always easy. I didn't have an international plan on my phone, so I called him every now and then from a call center. But, as every time we were separated by a trip, we emailed each other every day, religiously.

*   *   *

On Dec 21, 2013, at 10:38 PM, "Maria L. Sanchez Puerta" wrote:

hola osito!

how are you??

it was nice to see you briefly on skype today. I am at a bar trying to connect but the internet is pretty bad . . .

my mom brought my sister from bahía this afternoon. so nice to have vir here!!!

it seems like the internet connection on my mom's phone was super expensive so now she is not so keen on me using the whatsapp. and we will not have internet connection in the apartment until the 28. so from now on I might need to go to an internet café to get your news :(

how are you feeling? is your dad there already?

the kids are enjoying a lot. they really love the beach and are pretty comfortable in the water.

we miss you!

love you

lau

On Dec 22, 2013, at 8:45 PM, "Morgan" wrote:

Hola Lau,

it was nice seeing you on Skype as well, you looked great. How was your day today? Did the kids behave? Was it nice having Vir around?

My day was OK. I actually have not felt very nauseous today, which is unusual. My mom, dad and I got bagels in the morning. Then, my dad and I watched football while my mom went to see the movie Filamena, which she didn't like very much.

Anyway, I miss you,

Morgan

On Jan 8, 2014, at 1:34 PM, "Maria L. Sanchez Puerta" wrote:

hola Morgan

how are you feeling today? how did it go with the doctors?

what did they say about the lump? and about sex? ;)

hope all is going well!

we have gorgeous weather today! the kids had lots of fun in the sand. I will send you pics later today.

love you!!

Lau

On Jan 8, 2014, at 5:20 PM, "Morgan" wrote:

Hola Lau,

the appointments went really well, both doctors thought the lump had gotten significantly smaller. My infectious diseases doctor said my IV pump could come off in two weeks. Both doctors seemed to think the antibiotics were working well.

I feel pretty good today, very little nausea. I forgot to ask about sex, but that shouldn't be a problem.

The weather here has been brutal, incredibly cold. I read that in Chicago it was so cold that the zoo actually had to put its polar bear inside. I heard that buenos aires is having a heat wave, but that might be old news.

Julian will be 4 in two days, I can't believe he is that old. He is now a boy instead of a toddler. Anyway, I would like to skype with him on his birthday.

Kisses,

Morgan

* * *

Back in DC, we had a small domestic crisis. Rocío was very unhappy, complaining a lot about the children's behavior, about life, about her salary. She was skipping work a lot or bothering Morgan—who was in the middle of his recovery!—with requests to take her home after work because it was raining or cold.

I think one of the reasons for her dissatisfaction was that the kids were no longer babies, and she liked working with younger children. Julian had his own activities besides the Montessori preschool he was attending, and Clarita went two or three times a week to a different preschool. Both of them were starting to have activities that required moving them by car and Rocío did not drive. I decided to change our nanny mainly because of that. A cycle had come to an end.

That's how Maria came into our life and, still, as I write this, I cannot thank her enough for all the support she gave—and still gives—me in running the house and caring for the kids. Morgan had to go back to the hospital many times for the same symptoms: fever, nausea, infections. Many times I had to sleep there with him. Maria was a much-needed constant in the midst of so much uncertainty, helping us keep Julian and Clarita in their routine of school, swimming, and soccer. She was someone reliable who could stay over with them if I was forced to stay in Baltimore and their grandparents were not with us.

Beyond Morgan's recovery, which was progressing slowly, things seemed to be settling in pretty well. We had weathered the domestic transition from Rocío to Maria and I was able to travel to

Argentina in March and to Jordan in April for work. However, when I returned from Jordan, as if waiting for me, Morgan's back pain flared up again.

* * *

May 2014. We returned to Baltimore for checkups, and an MRI showed a result we hadn't expected. It wasn't certain, but among the scar tissue the doctors thought they saw a new tumor, the size of a small apple, that was pressing on the nerves and causing that excruciating pain.

Fear. Shock. I can't explain our feelings other than with those words. Dread overpowered us in an unstoppable wave. It swept Morgan back to his first painful operation before meeting me and to the nausea that caused him so much trouble. It forced me to confront my memories of the worst myxopapillary ependymoma prognoses that I had discovered the night of our first date, six years ago, and that I had decided never to look at again.

After that first rush of terror, we both looked to the future with more resolve than fear: we had to do all possible treatments. Besides, the doctors didn't know yet if it was the remainder of the tumor from the 2007 operation that was growing or if it was a new one, or how serious—or not—the matter was. I was scared about them opening his back again so soon, and scared he would have to go through the cycle of fevers, infections, pains . . . But I had to keep going. I was

Morgan's breadwinner. And I was not going to let him down.

* * *

Now I remember those days as a haze, where dates and moments blurred between comings and goings to Baltimore, waiting rooms, doctors coming and going, returning to our house, suddenly rushing to the hospital again for fevers that would not go down . . . because this second operation would only be the beginning of many more. In June, barely a month later, a third operation would be scheduled to clear the infection that had taken over the area after the second . . .

I see myself in the waiting room at Johns Hopkins, sometimes alone, sometimes with Morgan's mother or father, sometimes with my Uruguayan friends, Cecilia and Gabriel, so dear to me as almost siblings. Waiting . . . always waiting. I see myself putting together a little ritual to endure the hours of waiting: eating something delicious from Balducci's, watching a movie on my laptop while leaning back in an armchair in the waiting room, trying to distract myself. I see myself trying to keep a positive attitude, looking sideways every now and then at the screen with the patients' updates, waiting for the neurosurgeon, waiting for the plastic surgeon, waiting . . .

I am not the most empathetic person in the world. I rush to find solutions right away rather than dwell and complain. My way of persevering sometimes annoyed Morgan, who I never saw cry but who was heartbroken nonetheless. I learned the hard way over time not to propose fixes or plans right away—let's talk to the doctor, let's ask what you can take, let's do this, let's do that—but to let the other person simply unload.

But in May 2014 I still thought that a positive, proactive attitude was the most appropriate one, the one that could lead us to the other side of this trauma. I would suggest Morgan eat something he liked, or go out for some fresh air in the hospital garden. I wouldn't get upset and I didn't want anyone else to do so around Morgan, something that happened a lot when his mom was with him. Tamara and Nelson were a great help, and without them this stage would have been much worse. But Tamara was terrified, and it seemed to me that she contributed to the gloomy atmosphere.

"Morgan is depressed," she told me one day. *No. You depressed him*, I thought, although I didn't say it out loud. We had to get through this situation the best way we could, for the kids most of all. And I wanted to enjoy the moments with them and with Morgan as much as I could.

I would break down when no one could see me; neither Morgan nor the kids. I would cry both ways driving that hour back and forth between our house and the hospital, listening to Latin and romantic music on the radio. Songs that spoke of lovers who have to part, of loves that are no longer there. Like Christian Daniel's "Ahora que te vas":

The Word I Cannot Pronounce

Today I wake up with my soul in pieces
Today I say goodbye without wanting to say goodbye
Go slowly so I don't feel your footsteps
Go quietly so I don't hear your voice
I don't deny that I'm afraid
To face life without you
And now that you are leaving
You take my whole life with you
I don't even know where you'll go
But I understand that you'll have to leave
And now that you're leaving
Remember that love waits
And even if you never come back
I promise not to forget you
How can I forget you
I don't sleep alone, your portrait accompanies me
And in the mornings I usually appeal to God
That he no longer insists on tearing you from my arms
I'm already unable to bear so much pain
I don't deny that I'm afraid
Of facing life without you
And now that you're leaving
You take my whole life with you
I don't even know where you'll go

It was good for me to unload, but since I had to pay attention to my route, I was very efficient with my crying. I say that almost without irony.

* * *

"This operation unfortunately did not help," Dr. Goklasan told us. My head was spinning. They had taken out the tumor, they had operated again a month later to cure the cerebrospinal fluid infection that had formed in the wound, which was difficult to close, they had continued to puncture and drain it . . . and none of that had helped? Had the tumor grown again, in just a few weeks? It was all very confusing.

"We have to wait for the wound to close completely and try radiation for six weeks," said a specialist at Johns Hopkins. Now mid-July, it was already starting to get hot, and what in other years would have been a month of preparations for our summer vacation was now filled with preparations for a new treatment. In fact, for many months we had had tickets for an Alaskan cruise, one of Morgan's dreams. What were we going to do with those?

Morgan had already been treated with radiation in 2007, so the new dose was very low, with little margin for error, at a very delicate spinal site. And there was an additional concern. While the procedure was intended to stop the tumor from growing and killing all the nerves, making it difficult for Morgan to move, the radiation itself could induce peripheral neuropathy, meaning he might lose feeling in his right foot, the one most compromised by the tumor. In other words, the possibility of him losing mobility was now real.

Conversations began to get eerie. The operation to remove the tumor had not worked, the whole area was at risk of infection with each new operation, the tumor had come back, and with more force. We had entered another stage.

Tamara moved into the attic at home, where there is a bedroom and en suite bathroom. Every day for six weeks she drove Morgan to Baltimore for radiation. Morgan took a leave from his job, thanks to co-workers who donated their sick days so he could do the treatment without interruption. After those six weeks we waited impatiently for the radiation results, which wouldn't be clear until a couple of months after the treatment was over.

"I want you to go on the cruise," Morgan told me one day. I had tried to figure out how to get the four of us to go, plus my mom, who always came on vacation, but I didn't see that it was a wise thing to do this time. What if something happened in the middle of the cruise, an upset, a fever, an infection, in the middle of the ocean?

"I want you to go," he insisted. I finally acknowledged we all needed a break, and I knew Tamara would be staying with him. So we went. And upon our return, I pleaded with Morgan to come with us for a week to Sea Isle City, like every summer.

"Lau, I'm not going. I want to stay," he told me the day before we left. "You guys go and I'll join you later anyway."

"But no, how can you go alone, it's a four-hour drive! Let's go together. You don't have to be on the beach all day or socialize with my family or anyone else if you don't want to, or even leave the room. The house is huge, you can be alone as much as you want. Please come. It will be good for all of us."

Finally, I convinced him. He packed plenty of t-shirts to protect the radiation site from the sun—it couldn't be exposed at all—and he ended up having a good time with all of us, going into the sea, taking pictures, playing with the kids. Maybe the change of air loosened something in him. It certainly did in me. We were absolutely convinced, both of us, that the radiation had to have worked. We just had to be patient and wait.

* * *

October 2014. The office of Dr. Redmond, the radiation oncologist. I was already exasperated. A resident, with Morgan's chart in hand, told us that the radiation didn't work. The tumor did not shrink. It was still there, clinging to Morgan's back like a leech. At least that's what it looked like on the scans, tangled up and confusing among the scars. I kept calling it "tumor," I couldn't even pronounce the word "cancer." Morgan remained silent. I saw out of the corner of my eye that some tears began to flow behind his glasses. He tried to hold them back.

I couldn't hold back. I started asking one, two, ten questions that the resident couldn't or didn't know how to answer. The words seemed to resonate in a vacuum, to echo, to bounce off the walls.

* * *

The doctor finally arrived, but it didn't calm us down much. Everything was getting worse. Morgan was losing mobility. Still, I was determined to maintain a positive attitude.

"Are there any other patients, doctor, that have been able to go on with a normal life?" I wondered.

"Well, we have to see, it could be that, if it is the tumor, it grows very slowly . . . I have a patient who, wheelchair and all, continues to work and maintain his usual life," he answered.

"Can you give us their contact information? It helps us to know that others could do this."

The doctor also suggested inquiring about a chemotherapy protocol in New York. It was still experimental for treating myxopapillary ependymoma. We both said yes, excited to find something new to give us hope. We signed the papers and days later traveled together to New York to see Dr. Omuro, who led the experimental treatment.

"Anything that can be done, we'll do," Morgan said.

* * *

Checkups, checkups, checkups. Dr. Omuro, in New York, said Morgan would be a good candidate for the experimental treatment. Checkups, checkups, checkups, checkups. And a multi-page document requiring our consent: the side effects of the experimental treatment were so numerous that it would be better not to even think about it and just sign. What other option was left?

Some opt for alternative therapies, or to change their diet. In fact, Teresa, Morgan's sister, sent us books on nutrition and cancer. Other acquaintances told us about this or that healer.

However, both Morgan and I were always very practical. We trusted the medicine. Nothing alternative had been scientifically proven to cure anyone, his doctor told us. There is no proven connection between cancer and diet. And if on top of his illness Morgan had to give up meat or sweets, which were some of his few pleasures at this stage . . . he was not willing to lose them. The only dietary changes that we accepted, more as a new tradition than anything else, were the natural smoothies—kale, ginger, even chocolate—that Morgan's mother prepared every time he came home.

* * *

Checkups, checkups, checkups, and a new MRI so that we could start the new chemotherapy. This MRI showed that the tumor seemed to have shrunk minimally. Or at least it hadn't grown, which was good news. At a medical meeting, Morgan's doctors in

Baltimore decided that there was still some hope that inflammation and scar tissue were playing a role, that maybe the tumor wasn't growing.

So they recommended that Morgan begin steroid treatment without delay, to counteract the inflammation. I had to travel again, to Rwanda this time, and I heard the news in an email from him:

> Lau, a board of four neuro-oncologists, two radiation specialists and two neurosurgeons agreed that the problems I am having seem to be due more to the radiation than to the tumor growth. They think it would be a mistake to do the chemo and, instead, another round of steroids should be done. So I decided to go with them.

I wasn't too convinced. What's more, I was furious. Now the doctors had changed their minds, after having suggested chemo? Was there or wasn't there a tumor? Why was everything so confusing?

Meanwhile, new informed consent forms were arriving from New York detailing yet more new side effects that Morgan had to sign off on. We began to doubt the possibility of the experimental treatment as well.

"If I'm going to feel this bad with chemotherapy, I'd rather take the steroids and wait," Morgan told me.

A thousand questions spun through my mind as I anticipated possible futures. Morgan in a wheelchair, no sphincter control, unable to move? How were we going to manage it? Our house was full of stairs. Was Washington, DC a wheelchair friendly city? What were the streets like? I had never paid attention to these things before. Now, threatened by our possible new reality, I had to.

* * *

December 2014. A terrible year was coming to an end. The daily complications were many, the disappointments, too. But we were trying to get on with our lives, we loved each other, we loved the family we had created together. That the tumor—the cancer?—had broken into it made us cling even more to the little everyday pleasures while Morgan could still walk. Pleasures like a date at the Old Ebbit Grill—DC's oldest saloon and one of our favorite restaurants—or having sex again from time to time, despite the difficulties. Or for Morgan simply to be able to resume his work, or drive, or spend time with Phil, who needed support of his own after a car accident gave him a severe head injury he hadn't fully recovered from.

Steroid treatment began. Although Morgan was terribly bloated, the steroids also gave him energy and that had an impact on his mood, and mine. It didn't seem so far-fetched that I would travel back to Argentina with the kids, as I do every year, and Morgan could rest at home. We all needed to feel better. So we traveled. We would return on January 10, in time to celebrate Julian's fifth birthday together.

As I prepared for the trip, I recognized that this was our life now, with the good and the bad. I could not dither, bemoaning why we had to live this. I could not be bitter, railing against the gods or fate. To do so was to belittle everything we had, all our shared history. It's as Nina Riggs wrote in her cancer memoir *The Bright Hour*: "Thinking that way is like invalidating my life altogether. I have to love these days in the same way I love any other day. Maybe there's no such thing as 'normal' from here on out."

CHAPTER SEVEN

The Time of Uneasiness

"From one to ten, how much does it hurt?"

"Ten. I can't take any more pain," he answered. I froze. Morgan had never said anything like that to me before. He couldn't get out of bed. It was the night of January 10, 2015, Julian's birthday, and I had just returned from the annual trip to Argentina with the kids. It was as if Morgan's body had been waiting for our return to slacken and give in to the pain.

I immediately wrote to the neurosurgeon. The next morning, I went to our basement to get Morgan's walker. It had helped him years before, after the very first surgery, and he had brought it over from his previous home when we moved in together.

On January 23 we saw Dr. Gokaslan. I had emailed him some months earlier to thank him for all he had done for us. We really felt we were in good hands. He was gentle, considerate, warm. He was always willing to respond quickly, despite his position and duties. And he had always been so clear in his approach. It was the same this time.

"Morgan, the tumor continued to grow during this time. You may start to have sphincter problems and you will almost certainly lose the mobility of your right foot. There is no other option but to operate again to alleviate the pain and slow down the process."

So the year began with a new blow. The steroids, while they had given him energy, had also made his face swell terribly, and were no longer an option. In fact, they had accomplished nothing. A month wasted while the tumor continued to grow! Why hadn't we done the experimental treatment with chemotherapy? I felt guilty for not having insisted more, my head wouldn't stop, wouldn't stop, wouldn't stop. I didn't tell Morgan. He seemed calm about the decision: chemotherapy certainly had so many side effects and risks. We had done what we could. *Six months later Morgan would feel absolutely nothing from chest to toe. But we couldn't yet even imagine that.*

We decided the best thing to do was to try the operation and delay the cancer's growth as long as possible, as Dr. Gokaslan advised us. We had to make, in those first cold days of the year, another hard choice: Morgan retired on disability. Tamara helped us with all the paperwork. The focus now was on preserving as much of everyone's quality of life as possible.

"I'm a burden to you," he told me one day. "I should live somewhere else." He was having a hard time walking. I didn't feel any resentment and it hurt me that he thought so, but I tried to let him express his pain and fear however he needed to. It was not easy.

On January 30, he was operated on yet again at Johns Hopkins. Morgan's back had now undergone four surgeries and six weeks of radiation in less than two years.

*   *   *

Morgan had less and less mobility, less and less stamina. He was already in a motorized wheelchair for our walks around Arlington and our backyard games with the kids. The list of his medications was growing by the day. He had problems with blood pressure and blood clots. He had to do physical therapy to be able to walk at least once in a while.

"I don't want to live like this," he said one day, leaning on his walker. I tried to encourage him as much as possible, fighting my own hopelessness as I listened to him.

One afternoon he started feeling very dizzy. We called 911 and entered a circle of hell featuring three different hospitals in ten days, a spiking fever, and a new symptom: panic attacks. One night, I had gone out to dinner with a friend. Morgan came home from spending the evening with a friend of his own, felt his blood pressure dropping, and couldn't make it up the stairs to our room on the second floor. He didn't know what to do and started to get agitated. I raced back home to take him directly to Baltimore, terrified that the blood clots in his legs may have traveled to other parts of his body.

Like a wave that comes and goes, our equanimity returned as we returned home. At the end of March we even went out to celebrate my birthday, something that was always very important to me. Morgan knew that, and wanted to give me the pleasure. We went with Nelson, Tamara and the kids to a restaurant in Shirlington, one of Morgan's favorite neighborhoods. It wasn't an easy lunch; we were all pretty stressed out. Morgan had to shout for order: "It's Laura's birthday today, can everyone calm down a bit?"

Three days later, we were on our way to Baltimore again. He had to have his fifth operation. The wound in his back had become infected. He would barely leave the hospital again for several months.

* * *

This time, the incision would not close completely, and they had to apply a kind of vacuum-sealed sponge with a dressing to absorb the moisture. A machine attached to the sponge removed the draining fluids. During Morgan's brief stays at home over the course of those months, I would check almost obsessively that the machine was working properly, that the dressing was still sealed, because without that pressure the machine would stop working and the wound could become infected. My fear was that, if the device stops working, I wouldn't be able to fix the dressing and the nurses who had taught us how the device worked wouldn't arrive in time to keep infection at bay.

Keeping an eye on that device was one of a thousand daily worries, like remembering medications or soothing nausea, that left no time to think about other things. Managing the immediate, practical problems took away the anxiety of what might lie ahead and kept us focused on the present. This was our life now.

As he was trying to walk down the stairs at home one day, I heard Morgan yell to Tamara, who was helping him, "I'm scared to death!"

"But daddy, you're a big boy, how can you be scared? Shall I help you?" said Julian, who had heard. He kissed Morgan's cheek.

* * *

As Morgan essentially started living at Johns Hopkins, his parents and I took turns caring for him. I had started seeing a psychologist. What were we supposed to tell the kids? Was I doing the right things for them?

"The important thing is that they know what's going on," the psychologist told me. I needed to maintain their daily routine of going to school, continuing their activities. I tried to spend as much time as possible with them. I shuttled back and forth from my work to our house, from our house to the hospital. I stayed in contact with Morgan's doctors, checked on his medications and symptom changes, supervised the routine at home, updated the family with the latest news . . .

"Hi Laura, are you busy? Can I talk to you for a second?"

"Yeah, sure, Tamara, is everything okay? Is Morgan okay?"

That morning, Tamara called my office in Dupont Circle from the hospital. It was April 14. I remember it perfectly: a day before we had to send in our taxes, something Morgan had not yet taken care of for the year. I was reviewing reports and supervising my consultants on a World Bank project in Kenya.

"Laura, Morgan is talking nonsense."

"What do you mean, nonsense?"

"Something is wrong, Laura."

"Put him on." Morgan sounded delusional.

"I'll be right there," I told Tamara.

I alerted my boss. I called Maria to let her know I had to go to Baltimore urgently and ask her to please pick up the kids from school and stay with them until further notice, as I might not be coming home that night. I called my mom, my sister. I sent an urgent email to Dr. Gokaslan. I grabbed my wallet, cell phone charger, a couple of work folders and the car keys.

No thinking, no thinking. But I couldn't stop crying all the way from DC to Baltimore. I made it to the 12th floor of the hospital's Zayed Tower in record time. Morgan didn't recognize me, couldn't remember the children's names. He was babbling to Tamara about his past. He was taken to intensive care with a fever. I didn't go home. That night and the next few nights I spent in the hospital with Morgan. My mom started preparing for a trip to the United States to give me a hand. Nelson and Morgan's sister Teresa took emergency flights to Baltimore.

Morgan had had a cerebrovascular accident—a stroke.

*   *   *

Morgan was in intensive care for four days, slowly recovering in a totally isolated room. His weakened state, being sedentary, the constant operations, the medications . . . all had contributed to the small clot that had caused the stroke. He also had herpes zoster on his leg. I slept on a sleeper chair next to him. Teresa went to Target to buy me some clothes: pajamas, slippers, underwear. In the endless hours at the hospital those days, we felt very close to each other. My sister-in-law had traveled all the way from Phoenix thinking she might not get to see her brother alive.

Those were days of great anxiety. We didn't know if Morgan's symptoms were from possible meningitis or from the stroke. He was conscious but gone. He began to need diapers. The hours passed in scans and blood tests. Before this moment, my concern had been how to adapt our life to the fact that Morgan might not walk again. Now, in the intensive care unit, after the stroke, not knowing if he would be able to recover or not, I was no longer concerned about his mobility. I just wanted him to be lucid, for his mind to work well.

Unexpected resilience can arise in the face of extreme situations. I am an optimist by nature. And I think that, in those moments, instead of getting depressed, my body naturally produced the endorphins I needed to keep going. This let Morgan see me well. One day we put on some Latin music right there in the hospital room and Teresa and I started dancing. Morgan laughed. We were trying to put the best of our energy into a situation that was devastating us all.

Teresa's husband Daniel helped us file our taxes on time. From then on, he would help us with this kind of cumbersome paperwork many times. With Morgan's consent we transferred power of attorney to my name so I could take care of legal matters.

A week later, Morgan still couldn't remember our children's names, so I didn't want to take them for a visit and put everyone in a sad and uncomfortable situation.

"Daddy's in the hospital," I told them. "He's going to have to spend some more time there until he heals but we're going to go visit him on the weekends," I promised. I didn't know "some more time" would mean four more months.

Taking caregiving turns with Tamara and Nelson meant I could go back to the office and home, see Julian and Clarita, recharge my batteries. Morgan preferred to be with Nelson; he had a calmer character and helped Morgan distract himself, while Tamara spent her time fighting with the nurses, complaining if any medication was missing or they were late in attending to Morgan. It affected them both greatly to see their son declining, but Tamara was much more nervous.

Even though I wasn't the only one caring for Morgan, I was profoundly exhausted. A few weeks later, the possibility arose at work of a three-day trip to Milan with my boss's boss to present a report at an international NGO conference. It was several hours of work but, as was almost always the case on my trips, I would be able to make some time to walk around and distract myself. To have some free time, see Da Vinci's *The Last Supper* . . . it sounded wonderful. Nelson was in Baltimore taking care of Morgan, and my mom was in Washington, DC, which gave me peace of mind around the kids. I was on the verge of a breakdown, and I recognized that I needed to take care of myself a bit. So I agreed to travel.

* * *

The very first night, upon returning to the hotel, I had a message from the social worker who was handling Morgan's case at the hospital. She said Morgan had to leave Hopkins that week; his insurance wouldn't cover any more rehab. I couldn't believe they decided something like that when they knew I was out of the country for work; they all knew I wanted to be there if there was any change, let alone a transfer! I started calling his doctors, his father, everyone, desperate. Finally, we managed to postpone Morgan's discharge from the hospital until June.

When I returned from my trip, I had to start looking for a facility outside of Johns Hopkins where Morgan could continue intensive rehabilitation: occupational therapy, physical therapy, speech. In addition to the five different specialists we already consulted—his neurosurgeon, Dr. Gokaslan; his plastic surgeon, Dr. Sacks; his radiation oncologist, Dr. Redmond; an infectious disease expert, Dr. Kelly; and another oncologist, Dr. Holdhoff—we also started seeing a neurologist who oversaw all his various therapies. I wanted Morgan's rehab facility to be near the hospital. Dr. Gokaslan suggested instead that Morgan be closer to home to make his care more convenient for our family. But I preferred visiting Morgan in Baltimore to having him away from our most trusted doctor; easy access to Dr. Gokaslan gave me peace of mind.

The search was depressing. All I could find were nursing homes with a recovery wing, or places that considered Morgan's case was to be too complex, or not complex enough. I began to despair and to lobby the hospital to let Morgan stay in their rehabilitation center for a while longer. How could they let him go if his tests were bad, if the anticoagulants had to be closely monitored, if he could hardly move, if the fever came and went! With a lot of perseverance, insisting to doctors and hospital staff, I was able to extend his stay at Hopkins even longer.

At last, I found Future Care in Canton Harbor, a town very close to the hospital where several times I had gone with Nelson to eat vegan food, his favorite. They admitted Morgan on a Friday afternoon. However, the day we took him in, it turned out that the rehab center did not have the bare minimum needed for the treatment he required. They didn't have the necessary machine to absorb the fluids from the wound on his back, there was no device near the bed for Morgan to relieve himself, the bed had no rails . . . Tamara was helping me move him, and we both screamed our heads off about it.

It was already late at night. I had to go back to DC to take care of the kids because the nanny was finishing her shift. I texted the rehab doctor who had signed him out of Hopkins indicating that what they had done with Morgan was an unsafe discharge, they had forced him out of the hospital in a risky way.

"Bring him back!" he immediately replied . . . as if it were easy! Two women moving a six-foot-tall man who can't walk . . . And Morgan, exhausted, wanted to stay.

"Morgan, they don't have anything you need, we have to go back to Hopkins, I have all this weekend to find you a better place."

I convinced him without much trouble. It felt like part of a pattern I had begun noticing when he left intensive care to go to the hospital's specialized rehabilitation center. Something in his countenance made me think that his character was no longer the same. He was calm, very calm. Nothing seemed to bother him too much, nothing seemed to cheer him up too much. Considering everything that was going on, I thought maybe this change in his personality wasn't necessarily a bad thing.

* * *

A few days later I found Powerback, a rehabilitation center in Pikesville, Maryland, also near Hopkins. I worked hard to keep him in rehab there as long as possible—longer than anyone usually could in the United States—filing insurance paperwork to extend his stay so he could have around-the-clock skilled care. Morgan, however, wanted nothing more to do with the whole process. The rehabilitation exercises were tiring him out. He wanted to go home no matter what. I had a hard time convincing him that the longer he stayed at Powerback, the easier it would be to return home in better condition.

I also needed time to figure out how to get our house ready for him. I had a wooden ramp built from the garage to the basement. There we had a spacious room, with lots of light; it was the most accessible place in a house full of stairs. We could make it comfortable for Morgan. It could accommodate the bed that would be sent to us by insurance, as well as the machine to lift him, the IV stand and the intravenous medications. I would add in a television and an armchair for visitors.

His mother wanted me to put in an elevator chair to the dining room and another one to the second floor. It didn't seem practical to me. Getting in and out of those chairs, from there to the wheelchair . . . how were we going to do it without help considering how hard it was for him to move? I wanted to start with the simplest thing. Then we would see.

Besides, I had seen the elevator chair system at a neighbor's house. Her husband had used it during an illness. The man had died and the woman had been left with those chairs and that complicated locomotion device bolted to her house, like a reminder of her suffering embedded in the walls. I shivered just thinking about it.

Morgan's life at Powerback was a constant struggle. He complained every day about how demanding the place was. When I would go to talk to the director, he would tell me that, for example, Morgan had refused physical therapy that day, and if he kept refusing, he couldn't continue there. His case had too many complications: the clots, the sponge, the risk of infection, the current high blood pressure, the body that was beginning to deteriorate because it was not moving. We had already been told there was no possibility of continuing with the radiation. Physical therapy was the only thing, for the time being, that we could do to counteract the consequences of the tumor.

Then Dr. Gokaslan, whom I considered our port in the storm, wrote to tell us that he was moving to Princeton. I felt helpless: we had to change doctors. It was already July and my sister Vir was coming with her husband and baby daughter to visit me, as she did every year, for our annual planned vacation at Stone Harbor Beach in New Jersey. I was not sure whether to go or not. I saw Morgan more and more exhausted, and I was too. I visited him two or three times a week, and on weekends I took Julian and Clarita and we'd bring something delicious to eat or accompany Morgan to the facility's patio to get some air and a change of scenery. It had been a very difficult few months. Morgan insisted that we go to the beach for those five days of vacation. His parents would take turns taking care of him at Powerback.

Tamara was a lioness. Visitors were not allowed to stay overnight at the center, but she managed to get them to let her sleep on a mat next to her son. When Nelson replaced her, she stayed at a nearby hotel. I brought her a bicycle for the daily commute to Powerback.

Vir and I rented a van to travel to New Jersey from DC. As soon as we got in, I got a call from Tamara: Morgan's fever had spiked and he was being transferred to Hopkins. Again, I didn't know what to do. Was I getting out of the van? I started managing all the logistics over the phone. I wrote to Dr. Gokaslan who, even though he was already at Princeton, still had a lot of power at Hopkins. I was reassured that they were going to get him a room quickly. In a couple of days I would be back to take care of everything. I stayed in the van.

* * *

Metastasis. I got the news on the phone, in New Jersey, in a corner of the balcony of the apartment we had rented, where there was some signal. The tests he had undergone indicated that the cancer had spread to one of his vertebrae, the L3. They were considering a new operation. The doctor's words were bouncing around, echoing from one side of my mind to the other.

I knew that his back was unlikely to withstand further surgery. The wound would not be able to close. The antibiotics that would follow would make Morgan feel worse and worse. The options were few, one worse than the other. Morgan was going back to intensive care. I asked that he not have surgery until I returned.

I look back on those days now and can't believe a certain supernatural energy that happens to us, physically and psychologically, when we are cornered in a situation. How life goes on, takes over, in spite of everyone, in spite of everything. I see myself contorting to not lose the signal on that New Jersey balcony, talking to doctors and more doctors about the few options that could maintain a glimmer of health in Morgan. I remember going over and over with my sister and her husband the options that remained, if we would go back, if not. At least the kids enjoyed the beach and Clarita was able to celebrate her fourth birthday there.

We returned to Washington, DC the day after her birthday. We stopped by the hospital first. Morgan was in isolation in intensive care because of bacteria. We were able to get in with my sister, then she continued on to DC with my children. My mind couldn't stop scrolling through the possible options we had in the face of metastasis, that harsh word, carrying bad omens, that was sticking in my every thought.

Months earlier- thinking to treasure special moments- I had applied to an organization called Dream Foundation that granted last wishes to families dealing with cancer. We had been granted a trip to Disney World with the kids. But I saw we wouldn't be able to go after all. Morgan could no longer be away from the hospital.

* * *

A few days later, Morgan was finally moved from intensive care to a regular room. Dr. Holdhoff, the oncologist, asked me when we would all be in the room together—Nelson, Tamara, Morgan and me.

"Tomorrow," I said.

Every day we received bad news: he couldn't walk, stroke, meningitis, fever, infection, operations and operations, low blood pressure . . . what else could he tell us? It was July 7, 2015, six months into a year that had felt like a whole decade of weight on our backs.

CHAPTER EIGHT

Husband & Wife

On the afternoon of July 8, the first thing I noticed when Dr. Holdhoff, the oncologist, entered Morgan's hospital room was that he was accompanied by a doctor we had not seen before. Nelson, Tamara and I were sitting near Morgan's bed. Dr. Holdhoff had the latest tests in his hand. The results of the CT scan were a map of Morgan's whole body glowing phosphorescent yellow: one spot, the lungs; another spot, the hip.

"The analyses show that there is tumor activity in many places . . ." the doctor began.

It had happened. We had dismissed the possibility to the farthest corner of our thoughts during the previous months. But here it was. Dr. Holdhoff said, one by one, phrases that came like bullets. Metastasis. Nothing more to do. Maintain quality of life. Radiation so the hip won't break. Palliative care. Six months.

Six months. Time stood still. Tamara cried. Nelson cried. I cried as quietly as possible so as not to distress Morgan. The three of us could do nothing but sit, sit and cry.

Looking straight at Morgan, the doctor repeated: "You have six months to live."

On top of my shock and my tears, I was once again quietly grateful that after the stroke Morgan no longer took anything with either too much joy or too much sadness. Dr. Holdhoff and the other doctor, who had introduced himself as a palliative care specialist and was talking about wills and legal documents, were giving us the worst possible news. Yet Morgan's first response was to ask if he could do anything else to keep walking, what the radiation on his hip was like, how much he could receive. As if he didn't understand. Or as if he understood but still urged us to keep going.

* * *

I saved the dozens of questions that immediately formed in my head for when I could meet alone with Dr. Holdhoff. I didn't want to overwhelm Morgan or his parents, who were devastated. The palliative care doctor was fulfilling his role by telling Morgan not to worry, that they had everything he needed to be free of pain, that he would be comforted. But I needed to look closely at the tests and to have him explain what we could expect in the coming months. What it meant when Morgan went into palliative care. Whether he could come home. What documents we needed to prepare.

Within days, Nelson, Tamara and I dealt with Morgan's retirement savings, his life insurance. I signed a mountain of legal papers in my role as power of attorney. We considered Morgan's wishes for his last moments. Did he want to listen to music? Did he want to stay on a ventilator once there was nothing more to do? Did he want to be cremated or buried? Did he want people to visit him? What else did he want? I couldn't stop crying as I signed Morgan's name on one, five, ten documents. He remained calm.

It was all so unreal.

My best friend, Kiran, who lives in Boston, came to help me with the paperwork. We found out that I wouldn't be eligible for the Social Security Administration's widow's pension if Morgan and I were not married. That had never been an issue before; in fact, marriage had seemed like an unnecessary expense, an organizational mess. We didn't feel we needed it: we loved each other, what else was there? He was my husband, I was his wife, even if there was no paper to prove it. But now I was going to become solely responsible for the welfare of our children, and I would need all the financial help I could get. I also realized that I could add a special moment to our memories of each other. Neither of us had lost our sense of humor, nor the need for happiness in our lives.

And so I proposed to Morgan.

*   *   *

On Monday, July 20, I felt calm, in a good mood. I stopped by the Baltimore courthouse to pick up the necessary documents for the marriage. I wanted to propose to Morgan with the papers in hand. An officiant would be needed but it would be something simple, intimate. I wouldn't even take the kids, since it was a weekday and they had to go to school. I knew he would be happy about it.

When I arrived at Powerback, I met him in the rehab area.

"Morgan Dov Strasser, do you take Laura Sanchez Puerta to be your lawfully wedded wife?" I asked.

Morgan looked at me, smiled. And without any hesitation, he said yes. It made perfect sense to him. We couldn't talk much more at that moment, in the middle of the rehab room, but we agreed to have the ceremony a couple of days later, since, legally, we had to wait a day and a half until no one showed up to oppose our marriage.

Suddenly it seemed important to me that there were loved ones with us for the ceremony. I realized that even though it was happening under the most dire circumstances I could have imagined, it was our wedding, and was something to celebrate. Morgan's mother immediately offered to reserve a little room at Powerback. I began to think that his sister, Teresa, should be there, and maybe a couple of my friends as well. Teresa was immediately enthusiastic. She would travel from Phoenix with her husband and two sons, Nate and Andrew, and would be in charge of shooting a video and bringing some pizzas, the wedding cake, the music.

Nelson was already with us in Washington, DC. Kiran, who had returned to Boston, decided to come back. She would be in charge of finding both the flowers and an officiant who could come to the rehab center to marry us.

Like any bride, I was overcome with emotion. I decided to wear a cream-colored dress, with a flower print on the hem. I measured Morgan's ring finger to have some wedding rings made. I suggested to Morgan that he wear a white shirt that day, which he liked. I realized that Julian and Clarita had to be present at that important moment. Morgan had surprised me: even though he knew that, legally, this would make things easier for the kids and for me, he was really excited. In the midst of the pain, pleasure could appear, like lightning. Life continues to flow, even romance.

* * *

After work on Wednesday, July 22, I picked Kiran up from the airport, collected the kids, and drove us all to Baltimore. We arrived at six in the evening. At Powerback everyone was congratulating us, happy; you don't see things like that every day in such institutions.

I look back at the video that Teresa shot on her iPhone, which we later had edited with music, and I still get excited. We were, all of us, pure happiness, including Morgan. I put on my gold wedding ring.

Morgan's didn't fit—in the end his fingers were too swollen for him to wear it. We all talked, laughed, danced. Our family gathering transformed the atmosphere of a rehab ward into a celebration of life beyond circumstance. Tamara smiled as I had never seen her smile in those hard months, as I would never see her smile again. The kids played, ate lollipops. I hadn't told them that their dad and I were getting married; I didn't really know what to tell them, or how to explain that we hadn't been married before. So I told them something that was also true: that it was going to be a party. And it was.

"Do you take for your husband . . .?" the officiant began.

"Yes!" Clarita interrupted happily, before I could even open my mouth.

We all burst out laughing. Once we were declared husband and wife, Julian asked me if we were getting married.

I told him, "Yes, we are renewing our vows." I didn't want, at that moment, to give him a long explanation. Since then, they have both always said that their parents "married twice." We managed to build, among all of us, a beautiful, indestructible memory of our family and our love.

* * *

After a few bouts of fever and radiation sessions on his hip, on August 21 Morgan finally returned home. He wanted quiet and to be with the kids. My friend Carolina organized a Meal Train: different friends, on stipulated days, would bring us homemade meals for Morgan to enjoy so that we wouldn't have to spend as much time dealing with food.

The bright room in the basement was ready with everything we needed. Besides the odd checkup or adjustment, Morgan would no longer have a swarm of doctors around. That was my only consolation. Basically, all that was left was to manage his pain. He didn't have to take any more medications, except for blood thinners and antibiotics. A nurse came by once a week to check everything. We were calm. Morgan knew that I would always be by his side, unconditionally. And he, because of his temperament, often preferred to be alone than to have a crowd around him; the quiet of our home suited him.

Visits from his parents became less frequent. Tamara started having some health problems of her own, including very painful urinary tract infections. She also suffered a lot from seeing her son in decline. In November Nelson would be diagnosed with lymphatic cancer and would have to have chemotherapy. Since he had been an athletic and healthy man all his life, he was able to handle the treatment well, and between sessions he would come to see Morgan.

Our routine changed, of course. I took care of all the daily logistics. Morgan slept with a little bell by his side so he could call me at any time. At first, I would come down at night to check that everything was okay, like a mother does with a newborn. I soon realized that Morgan slept peacefully through the night.

In the morning, as soon as I woke up, I would set up the catheter, empty the urine bag, get him ready for the day. Maria, our nanny, would bring him breakfast while the kids got ready for school and came down to give him a kiss. Before I left for work, the first big shift of the day was to move him from the hospital bed we had been given by the insurance company to a recliner, so he would be more comfortable and could be distracted by the TV. Upon my return from work, we would go out in the wheelchair to walk with the kids, or they would stay and play in the basement. Three times a week, a hospice caregiver came to help us bathe Morgan in bed.

On a small table were his medications; in another corner, a portable toilet and a walker, with which for a while he tried to continue the therapy he had done at Powerback. But that didn't last long. He could no longer feel his right foot, which was supported by a kind of metal boot. With that boot, Morgan could move from the bed, leaning on the walker, take a step, sit up, and be able to manage his foot. But his feet were swollen, so fitting them into the boot and slippers so that he could go to the bathroom or sit in the wheelchair was an almost torturous procedure. It wasn't long before he started wearing diapers and an indwelling catheter for urine.

Once, while I was trying to help him stand up, his legs gave out and he fell next to the bed. I started yelling in desperation to Maria and Tamara—who was still visiting us at the time—to get them to come down. I don't know how, but between the three of us we managed to lay him down. It was already evident that standing up was bringing more problems than benefits. Near the end of September, when he truly couldn't stand anymore, we installed a hoyer lift, a mechanical device to lift him out of bed and move him to the couch.

On September 24, we celebrated Morgan's 47th birthday with the children and Morgan's friends Phil and Mike. Morgan was on the couch, happy with the visitors, with the candles on the cake, with the singing, and above all for something we never stopped doing: taking advantage of the opportunities for celebration that life still gave us, even if they were few. In the photos of that day, Julian and Clarita are radiant, and I am smiling. The four of us wear little birthday hats. Our joy is so genuine that sometimes when I look at those pictures, I forget the difficult situation we were going through.

Finally, around this time, doctors took out the machine that absorbed the fluids from the sponge in the wound on his back. Now it had to be covered with gauze that needed to be changed regularly. Once a week hospice came to put special patches on it, but I took care of the day-to-day. I bought him a mattress that inflated and deflated in different parts and I changed its position every night to avoid bedsores caused by immobility.

It was very reassuring to talk to Juan Carlos, a friend's husband who is a doctor. With a lot of patience, he explained details to me, gave me perspective, and told me how the situation would deteriorate so that I could feel prepared. And he made useful practical suggestions, too. He suggested, for example, that I ask to switch to an anticoagulant that was easier to dose and monitor; the change took a huge weight off my shoulders. He also helped me think through which medications could be pared back so we wouldn't be quite as burdened by the extensive regimen that was no longer offering meaningful benefits.

The pain, that companion that would not leave our side, became more and more intolerable. Morgan was losing feeling in his legs and the pain was taking over. His remaining medications made him both nauseous and constipated. Then he began having difficulty breathing, due to clots in his lungs. Soon he got bedsores from always lying down, despite my special mattress and care.

"It is not possible to stop the damage, Laura. It will progress no matter what you do," Juan Carlos told me.

I watched Morgan deteriorate a little every day. But we kept going.

* * *

I was very worried about the children. We had not yet talked about the fact that their father was only going to be with us for a little while longer, about death. They were so young! Even I still had a hard time digesting the word "cancer" at that point. My friend Kiran sent me a link from the American Cancer Society about how to talk about death to children of different ages. I also consulted with an educational psychologist and the social workers at the hospital. How do you explain to two children, four and five years old, that their father is going to die?

Morgan and I decided to talk to them together, using simple words. I wrote several drafts, trying different ways to tell them something so sad and so difficult. Morgan chose which part to say himself. We practiced a bit.

Finally, we sat down to talk to them one Sunday night. It was September 7. The next day, school was starting. In fact, Clarita was changing to the Montessori preschool, and Julian was starting kindergarten. Today I wonder why we chose such a day, with so many changes looming for the kids. I don't know. The weeks before, with Morgan's arrival home, we had been adjusting to the new routine. And, in the very uncertain circumstances we were in, where anything could happen suddenly, we really couldn't find a better time.

We were in Morgan's room, playing with them.

"Guys, we wanted to know how you are," I told them in English, the language the four of us used to communicate, although when I was alone with them I spoke to them, and still speak to them, in Spanish. "Do you guys understand what's going on with Papi?"

That's how the talk began. We told them that it had been two years since Daddy had been sick, that the doctors and the hospitals, all of them, had done their best to cure him. However, the remedies and treatments had not worked. Daddy's illness could not be cured. So, when something like this happens, the body stops working.

"I'm going to die," Morgan told them. "We don't quite know when it's going to happen but we're going to be at home, facing this together."

"Daddy's not going to be in pain and he is going to be very comfortable," I added. "This is no one's fault. People die, some sooner and some later, but what we feel for each other doesn't die."

"Daddy, are you going to die?" said Julian.

"Yes. Sometimes people who get sick, we die. But that doesn't always happen, almost all people live for many years."

Julian and Clarita looked at each other and, after a while, they were playing again. They asked no more questions. I was in shock, Morgan calmer. We were both relieved: we had had a chance to talk. It had been a huge burden to plan that talk, the hardest I'd had with our kids in a long time. Both Morgan and I thought we had taken a big step. I didn't yet know the questions, emotions and reactions the kids would have later, when there was no time to prepare my responses.

After that we started reading books to them that would help them better understand the situation. Children's books like *The Invisible String*, *Wherever You Are: My Love Will Find You*, and *Lifetimes*, which talk about how long living beings live or how people who love each other stay connected despite everything. I wanted them to understand the idea that once Morgan died, he was not going to be with us anymore except in our hearts. And I told them that dying from an illness like their dad, or in a car accident like their grandfather, was an exception to the usual. I didn't want them to be afraid that something was going to happen to them or to think that we were all going to die soon or to feel guilt. I recorded Morgan reading some children's goodnight stories to them, so they would have a memory just for them.

I also decided therapy could help them, and help me support them. They started doing art therapy at a center called Life With Cancer. Clara talked a lot there, expressing herself. Julian, quieter by nature, not so much. As for me, I think I lived with my adrenaline constantly pumping, solving daily issues. My psychologist, who was also director of counseling at the World Bank, always deliberately told me to be careful, that I could get very low once the adrenaline stopped its frenetic pumping in my body.

* * *

By October, Morgan's pain was increasing yet again. The tumor was growing, pressing on his nerves, paralyzing him. Despite that, we were still trying to lead as close to a normal life as possible: going out with the kids for a walk or the two of us going to the movies together. Getting out was a logistical nightmare involving the hoyer lift and taxis with built-in ramps, but it was worth it; I remember how much Morgan loved *Mission Impossible*. At home we'd watch television series like *The Big Bang Theory* or *How I Met Your Mother* on our iPad. Teresa traveled a couple of times from Phoenix to see us.

Teresa was well aware of Morgan's pain, and even once paid for a visit from an acupuncturist in case they could help Morgan's suffering. A very Zen-like lady came to our basement. She succeeded, momentarily, in relieving Morgan's pain, but not for long. He did not want to try this therapy again.

He also didn't like talking to the chaplain, a spiritual counselor sent by hospice. I used to sit in on some of the conversations. We would talk about practical things—she suggested activities to do with the kids, for example—and about our feelings. It was a relief for me to talk to her. Morgan, however, preferred to be left mostly alone. He wanted to be with me or the kids, but not for very long, because even our company tired him out. He read, he watched TV, he slept. He slept more and more.

On October 11, he was in so much pain that we had to call an ambulance to take him to a hospice in Aldie, Virginia, where he was hospitalized. They put a little device on him that he could squeeze during the pain and the pain medicine would go straight to his blood. Soon afterwards he lost all feeling from the chest down.

In the meantime, between all these profound changes and people passing by the house day after day, the kids became more and more rebellious. They wouldn't listen to me, they fought with each other, and they both came into my bed at night, which they had never done before. I was so overloaded. Sometimes I felt like I was going to disappear, pulled apart in a thousand directions.

At the end of October, we shot a legacy video. I wanted the kids to have a testimony of their dad, of what his life had been like, told by him, for when they grew up and had questions. Morgan agreed. Teresa organized a Skype interview with the nonprofit Thru My Eyes. The interviewer asked Morgan questions and he recounted his life: his childhood in California, his travels, his studies, his interests, his work. His favorite color (blue), his favorite foods (sushi, roast beef), his best memories (when he found out about my pregnancies, his graduation day, our wedding). I was happy to see that there were few things about Morgan's life that I didn't know. That meant that we had talked a lot in all these years together.

At the end of the video, I also appear, next to him, talking about us and our children. Morgan lights up when talking about them. He defines Clarita as a beautiful baby, always happy, laughing, singing. Julian as a bundle of energy, sweet, athletic, strong. He says he loves that they sit on his lap and let him read them stories, that they are always hovering around him, even if it's just to see what the nurses are doing.

The best thing about being a parent, Morgan says in the video, is watching them grow up: watching Julian play sports, Clarita dance.

"I hope they've learned from me to be trustworthy, to not lose their temper, to be able to face whatever they go through with maturity, to be gentle with people. What did I learn from them? I learned to be more mature, to not stress so much."

"Anything else you'd like to add?" asks the interviewer at the end of the video.

"This is for Julian and Clarita. I hope that, if I'm not with you to see it, you have a good life, you do well in your studies, you have beautiful relationships. That's the important thing. That's all."

* * *

November came with the cold that heralded, in more ways than one, the winter to come, but we managed to have some good times and get out of the house a bit, like the day we went to see an NBA game. My cousin Pepe, the basketball player, had not only gotten us tickets to a game but had arranged for Manu Ginóbili, the Argentinian star of the team, to come and greet us.

I arranged for a cab to take us and wait for us. When we arrived we realized that Manu wouldn't see us until the end of the very long game. We ate donuts and drank hot tea to hold us until the end. We enjoyed it even though I was very worried: was Morgan feeling well, wasn't he tired? I still can't believe that, with him in his condition, we were sitting there just like the many thousands of other people who filled the stadium. I planned these special outings, even though they were so difficult, because I wanted him to have exciting things to look forward to in whatever time he had left to live. I wanted to treasure exceptional moments with him so he could take those memories with him, and so I could keep them myself.

Finally, passes in hand, we waited for Manu Ginóbili backstage. He greeted us very kindly, and we took pictures. A week later, we repeated the scene but with the actor Ethan Hawke, of whom we were both fans. He was coming to a Washington, DC synagogue to present his third book, a sort of compilation of maxims for his children.

Again, I arranged for us to be driven and waited for during the event. We were in the front row. I had talked to the organizers to try to get Morgan a chance to say hello. However, I had only wrung from them a promise that Hawke would sign a book for us and no certainty of being able to greet him. At the end of the presentation, the wheelchair-accessible route took us out a back door and Hawke came out that way, too. He spoke with us warmly and agreed to a picture.

Teresa suggested we see the *Avenue Q* musical, a puppet show for adults. It was playing at the Constellation Theater, a small venue I had never heard of. By intermission I saw that Morgan's energy was flagging, and I asked him if he wanted to stay for the second part.

"How interested are you in the show?" he wondered.

"Very interested."

"Okay, then we'll stay."

It was a very nice gesture on his part. He was sick, but in our pairing, I still mattered too.

The next day, Morgan woke up very weak. His hemoglobin, which we measured frequently and should have been around 9, was at 3. I had to take him to Sibley Hospital, where the kids had been born, for a blood transfusion. At the hospital, as soon as we arrived, his hemoglobin measured at 9. It had been a mistake in the previous measurement, which the nurse had done at home. We never knew why. Nelson, who was visiting, stayed overnight with him. And I couldn't believe what had happened. It was one thing to make the effort to take him out of the house to do some activity with the two of us together or to go for a walk with the kids, as we would go days later to the opening of MOM'S, an organic store near our home. It was quite another getting him out of bed in the middle of the night, my heart in my mouth, to take him to the hospital.

Thanksgiving came, another nice time to treasure. Morgan's best friend Phil and his wife Reut came, as did our former nanny, Rocío, and her son. Strangely—and wonderfully—we were also joined by the actress Tiana Alexandra-Silliphant, whom I had met a couple of days earlier in the café at the Tabard Inn, a hotel across the street from my work. I was there with a friend and she overheard us talking and joined us, sharing that her husband, screenwriter Stirling Silliphant, had died of cancer years before. On an impulse, I invited her to our dinner.

Morgan was hospitalized again shortly before the meal and I called Tiana to let her know we might have to cancel. And she came to the hospital to see us! Morgan wanted to kill me. He didn't want anything to do with strangers hanging around. The actress ended up chatting with Nelson in the waiting room. Morgan came home in time for us to make Thanksgiving dinner.

By then, I knew he had only a few weeks to live. He was very pale and thin. I could not just collect beautiful family memories; I had to confront our painful reality. How was I to know if he was dying, what was I to do, how was he to bear it, how was I to bear it? Really: how was I to bear it? I had many talks with the social worker about the ways in which people could die, trying to minimize the inevitable panic.

My friend Kiran, always willing to help me, began to look with me at what options we had, in the state of Virginia, regarding cremation and funeral services. It involved so much paperwork that it was not something I could leave to the end. I also thought anew about the ceremony I could have to honor him at his death.

It was hard to think of things like that with Morgan still alive, but someone had to do it. Neither Tamara nor Nelson wanted to hear anything about it. Morgan's mom didn't even want to come to Washington, DC for any ceremony we might have. I asked Teresa for help—could we figure out together what to do for it? She wrote me back quickly and said she couldn't think about it, it was too much for her.

It was all too much for me, too. I felt very lonely.

CHAPTER NINE

On That Day

The year seemed reluctant to come to an end. November, despite the occasional cool day, was still sunny and warm, and we could still make plans as a family: not only Morgan and I alone, but also with the kids.

A doctor still came once a week to check on his health. I always had questions. Somehow I thought that, by staying on top of the facts, I could make things flow better for all of us. I wanted the doctor to give me an idea of how much longer we had left, how the progression of the disease was going to go.

At the beginning of the month, Morgan still had the capacity for enjoyment and that was a relief to me. He enjoyed the food, which kept coming through the Meal Train from our friends, he enjoyed our outings, reading, watching movies with the kids. I also enjoyed riding with Morgan on the wheelchair while the kids rode their bikes: we would go out to the back street behind our house, a very quiet little internal street, and Morgan would organize races in his chair, with Julian and Clarita each on their bike or sitting on top of him. He was going at a speed that scared me!

In order for Morgan to get out, even for a few minutes, we had to help him get dressed, comb his hair, cover the catheter, put him in the chair. It was quite a production. But it was worth it. The shouts of happiness from the kids and Morgan's pale face turning color, flushed by the speed and the fresh air, made me feel happy. Even if only for a few moments, it was like catching up on old times.

* * *

However, the colder days that began to arrive in December, heralding the snowfall and sub-zero temperatures of an approaching winter, brought other signs as well.

Morgan started sleeping more, eating less. I forced him to take a protein shake at least twice a day, even if he didn't feel like it, so he could stay hydrated and minimally nourished. After each day, each with its own complications, in the evenings we would relax by watching TV after the kids were asleep, usually romantic comedies or series about lawyers and politicians like *Suits*, *House of Cards*, *Scandal*, and *Homeland*. Morgan in his bed, me on the couch next to him. I would put the iPad with that night's series on a small high table, where he had his medicines and always a bottle of water. Our watching also filled the time he needed to get the intravenous dose of one of the daily antibiotics; it took two hours to come down.

One night in early December, when the kids were asleep and we were watching *Suits* together, I noticed that Morgan was no longer following the plot. We always commented on the twists and made predictions about what might happen, but that night, when I asked him what had happened in a scene we had just seen, he couldn't say the names of the characters.

I let it go; I didn't want him to feel bad. But I realized it wasn't just a lack of concentration. He was losing his cognitive function, having trouble stringing sentences together. It was one of the signs I'd been looking out for. So was the morning when he woke up and started calling for his mother as if he had just returned from riding his bike with her, as if he was still a child. He was not aware that it had been a dream.

From that moment on, I would not be sure when he was fully lucid and when he was not. I started to feel really afraid of his impending death. Morgan didn't talk about it. He had always been very private about his feelings, and after the stroke, even more so. He focused on the day to day because he wanted to be well. That focus gave us both a way to keep going.

I was used to his physique deteriorating. Because of his youth, the damage had been gradual. We had been able to adapt little by little, and he was stoic despite the intense pain. But what would happen when his mind no longer responded? When his clarity, his intelligence, his way of analyzing and describing things would disappear? Would he still be Morgan?

* * *

I had no trouble talking about what was happening. It was my life, my daily reality. I kept leaning on my psychologist, my family, my friends. Most people find it difficult to talk about these issues, though, so nobody knew very well what to tell me, how to comfort me, what to ask. I released a lot on my own, by crying. It was my "efficient" way of letting go of all the feelings, the sadness and fears I had, as it had been when Morgan was hospitalized at Hopkins and I would take advantage of the hour drive from Washington, DC to cry.

I resolved not to let go of the little things that made me feel good. Christmas was approaching, perhaps the saddest of all because I knew it was our last with Morgan, and I started making cards for all the people who had helped us in that difficult 2015: nurses, friends, Hopkins staff. I would add a chocolate or some candy to the envelope. It was another kind of therapy.

In mid-December my mom arrived for a month. It was a relief and a support for me, who already had to face alone, and without further delay, the fact of organizing the ceremony to remember and pay tribute to Morgan when he was no longer with us. I didn't tell him much about it; that aspect *was* very difficult to talk about. At some point we touched on it in a very short conversation. He told me he wanted something intimate, at home. At home as he had always liked to be.

Teresa also came to visit us in mid-December, for three days. One night we went together to buy Ensure, the protein shake Morgan needed and had run out of. We stopped for coffee at a Starbucks. She offered encouragement about the kids and Julian's rebellious behavior, told me memories of Morgan. She thanked me for my care and said she had always admired so much the love we had for each other, how we laughed together even in the worst of times. Since that time at Hopkins when Morgan suffered the stroke and she flew to see him, I had felt closer and closer to her. Teresa said I was the sister she didn't have. I was so glad she was happy that Morgan and I had found each other.

* * *

We celebrated Christmas at home with my mom, Phil and his wife, and our kids. We made a lovely dinner and Santa Claus brought presents for Julian and Clarita in the morning. From that point on, Morgan's physical deterioration was noticeable. He hardly spoke at all. One day he had diarrhea, the other a fever . . . The new year arrived and my main concern became making sure the children did not lose contact with their father, nor he with them. Morgan was very weak and could no longer play. There were no more wheelchair races or stories in the evenings.

We started watching movies from the '80s together as a family, the ones that had marked Morgan's and my childhood and adolescence: *Back to the Future*, *Karate Kid*, *The Neverending Story*, *E.T.* Every night the four of us would watch one together and eat pizza or something else tasty. Morgan would fall asleep during most of the movie but it was still something we could share. Nelson and my mom, who were both with us, often joined us.

They both stayed until January 11, the day after Julian's sixth birthday. I wanted my oldest son to have his celebration in spite of everything, so he could remember a happy moment. So while Nelson took care of Morgan, my mom helped me organize the birthday at an event hall. Kiran sent from Boston some party favors for Julian's little friends. When we got home, the four of us took a picture. It is our last picture together.

* * *

When Nelson and my mom left, I realized I was on my own for the end. I didn't know how Morgan was going to die or how I was going to react. I needed help so the kids could get on with their lives. I arranged for Maria or a neighbor to stay with Morgan when the kids needed to be taken somewhere or I needed to stop by the office for a while.

On January 14, Morgan started having mild delirium. He recognized me, he recognized the kids, but he could no longer carry a conversation. Then he started sleeping most of the day. These were more signs that his body was shutting down, that he was ceasing to be a part of this world. But I felt calm. Once or twice a week the nurse would come to bathe him or the social worker would come to check how everything was going and I would take the opportunity to ask them what to expect in the days to come.

On the morning of January 20, when I went down to the basement to see him, the scene was different from every other morning. Morgan was very sweaty, his water bottle was knocked over, the sheets were disheveled. He was breathing heavily. He wasn't talking. I called the doctor, who told me it was time to start him on liquid morphine, to calm him down. The kids went down to the basement to greet him before leaving for school and noticed immediately that he was having trouble breathing.

"Daddy is not very well. But don't worry, he's not in any pain," I assured them.

They had never seen him like this before and were scared. I told them I would not go to work. Later I learned that Clarita cried all day at school.

* * *

"I'm scared," Morgan said, squeezing my hand. The morphine had calmed his body and he was lucid.

"What are you afraid of, my love?"

"Of death."

I didn't know what to tell him, I had a lump in my throat. Then I remembered a book Teresa had sent me: *Final Gifts*, by Maggie Callanan and Patricia Kelley. It's about the needs of dying people, their special state of care and communication about what is happening to them. The book had testimonials from people who had been on that passage to death but had survived to tell the tale: they all spoke of a peaceful passage, without suffering.

"Do you want me to read you something from this book? You will like it."

I showed it to him. He nodded. I read about the light that accompanied that transition to another stage.

"Many dying people see a place not visible to others. Their descriptions are short and not very specific, but in general they speak of light and radiance. They all describe the place as beautiful." I saw that he was being soothed.

In another excerpt I read to him, the authors agreed that this "other place" people see is a sign of a life beyond death. A paradise, for those who believe in it, though even those who do not profess any religion describe it that way. Something as beautiful and pleasant as a dream but with the certainty that it is real.

I also calmed down. I had to make an enormous effort, perhaps the greatest so far, not to cry inconsolably when he asked me:

"Am I going home?"

*   *   *

I played music for him, turned on the TV. A nurse came to see him and told me that Morgan might be able to stay with us for a few more days, maybe a week.

He prescribed another medicine to help Morgan breathe better. I thought Morgan wouldn't be alive even that much longer, but I knew we should still go through the daily routine. I had to pick up the medicine from the pharmacy and the kids from school. I asked hospice to send someone that afternoon to stay with Morgan for an hour while I picked up Julian and Maria, the nanny, picked up Clarita.

When we returned home, Morgan was sleeping soundly, one of the effects of the morphine. The kids saw him and went upstairs with the nanny. I stayed next to Morgan, along with the person hospice had sent. For a minute—eternal for me—I noticed that he stopped breathing, then caught his breath and started up again. I looked at the man.

"This happened while I was gone? What does it mean?"

"Better call hospice, ma'am. It's getting close."

Our social worker and the nurse who had been with us the last few times came within minutes. The man left. They stayed by my side until Morgan took his last breath. He seemed at peace. In the quiet of the room, in front of other people, although it gave me peace to be accompanied, I preferred not to speak aloud. I love you, I said in my thoughts, to say goodbye. At half past five in the afternoon of that freezing January 20, Morgan died.

* * *

The world and time stopped. Everything stopped spinning. Ceased to exist. There was only that room, that cold afternoon, Morgan as calm in bed as if he were asleep, his features relaxed. The moment I had so dreaded had arrived. I felt a strange calm. I knew I had done everything in my power to see that he lived in the best possible conditions for as long as possible. We had both done everything to stay together, to live our lives.

I stayed in the room for a while, next to the social worker and the nurse who gently told me that cremation services needed to be called. I wanted a few minutes alone with Morgan. I lay down next to him. They would come for his body in the evening.

After some time with Morgan, I knew I had to go upstairs to the kitchen.

The kids had already changed and eaten dinner, and were with Maria. Daddy died, I told them, simply. Somehow, despite their age, they already knew it was going to happen, and seeing him that morning before school had given them a clue that something was going to change immediately. Did they want to see him? Julian immediately said yes. I could see that Clarita was not sure but, as her brother said yes, she also agreed.

The nurses stayed a while longer. Then Joanna arrived, a friend who, in the previous days, I had invited to dinner. I let her know that Morgan had died and she asked me if I wanted her to stay anyway. I said yes. I needed company. Then my best Argentinian friend in DC, Alexandra, arrived. Phil arrived. The nurse and the social worker left.

We went down to the basement with the kids. Clarita slowed down at the entrance when she saw Morgan in his bed, inert; she was a little scared.

"I'd rather send him a kiss from here," she told me.

That was her way of saying goodbye and having a memory, a closure with her dad. Julian, on the other hand, went straight to Morgan's bed and climbed on top of it. He stood on his pillow, climbed up on the hoyer lift like he used to, like a little monkey.

A while later we went upstairs and I let Phil, who had been attached to Morgan since he was so young, have a quiet goodbye to his best friend. I started making the necessary calls: to Nelson, to Tamara, to Teresa, to my family.

It was already close to nine o'clock at night and I accompanied the kids to their room. I told them that they were taking Dad with them, too. They already knew that, from now on, he would no longer be at home but that they would always carry him in their hearts.

My two friends stayed and we had dinner together. We drank wine. I was very calm. Heavy snow started to fall against the windows. We tried to relax as we waited for the cremation service to come get Morgan's body. Because of the storm, they didn't get to the house until 11:30 p.m.

I watched Morgan leave on a stretcher, just like the many recent times we had had to rush him to the hospital. It was exactly the same. He looked asleep and I couldn't believe that, this time, he was being taken away from home for good, in the middle of the snow.

Joanna left. Alexandra stayed overnight to keep us company. I climbed into bed and fell fast asleep, exhausted, as the storm raged outside. Perhaps that deep sleep was part of the almost surreal feeling of having watched the love of my life die. It may seem strange, but I didn't feel alone. He was somehow still with me.

* * *

The next day, Nelson, Teresa, and her husband arrived. We agreed to have an intimate ceremony at home the following day, January 22: us; Phil and Reut; and my cousin and his wife, who would travel from Detroit on behalf of my family, since neither my mom nor my sister could travel in time. Outside, it snowed relentlessly. Some friends who wanted to stop by to say hello could not make it because of the mountains of snow accumulating in the streets.

I didn't want to hold a gathering in the building where the cremation takes place. It didn't seem good for the kids nor did I like the impersonal setting. Nor did I want a funeral like you see in the movies. I wanted something quiet, as Morgan said he wanted.

To alert the rest of our friends and acquaintances, I had prepared, together with Kiran, a website with photos of Morgan. We included a eulogy that Teresa wrote to share a bit about who he had been and what he liked. She mentioned his favorite movies, including *As Good As It Gets*, starring Jack Nicholson.

She wrote: "As the hero of this movie says, 'You make me want to be a better person.' And Morgan had that effect on many of us who knew him, challenging us to match his gentleness, his openness, his kindness and his generosity of spirit. He spent his last days with his wife and children, smart and funny to the end."

On the website we warned the ceremony would be very small and private but we would be available a few days later to receive anyone who wanted to stop by the house to greet us. Our doors would be open. Instead of flowers, we suggested donations to the American Cancer Association and Life With Cancer, organizations that had helped us so much.

I posted the link to my Facebook page. I received hundreds of messages through the website and Facebook, dozens of emails as well. They all talked about what a great person Morgan had been and shared memories. Teresa wrote a very beautiful post about her brother, highlighting his kindness, his sense of justice, his transparency, how much he loved Julian and Clarita. It touched me. It was a comfort to feel so fully the warmth of those who appreciated us, to remember once again—because I already knew it—that Morgan had been so loved.

* * *

At noon on the 22nd, Tamara connected via Skype. She could not bear to be present at the ceremony in person. It was very hard for her emotionally and, besides, she was very sick. We didn't know it yet, but she also had cancer, a disease that seemed to haunt us.

My mom and sister also connected via Skype. Morgan's best friends, Phil and Mike, and two couples friends of ours came to the house, as well as the hospice nurse who had been with us several times, the social worker, and the chaplain, whom I had asked to help us conduct the ceremony. She helped me select two poems, one to be read by me, one to be read by my cousin.

I wanted to film a video of the ceremony but Teresa asked that we not. Because of her work in television, she would not be able to be calm or cry if we filmed something that could become public. I understood.

We gathered in the living room of our house. On one table, bagels and coffee. On another, photos of Morgan that Teresa had enlarged, some candles, and three plugged-in iPads connecting Tamara, my mom, and my sister to the event. We set out a container in which each of us would place a small transparent stone while sharing a memory about Morgan. It was something simple and emotional that Julian and Clarita could also participate in.

I couldn't help but start crying as soon as I uttered the first words of the poem—some verses by James Miller, a contemporary poet—that I had chosen to pay tribute to my husband and, with him, to our love and our family:

Death means nothing
I just slipped into the other room
I am me and you are you
What we were to each other
That we still are

Call me by my old name
Speak to me in the old way . . .

It was the first time, in all this time, that the kids had actually seen me cry. I spoke about the moment Morgan and I met, right on time, my favorite story about the two of us. I spoke about Morgan's honesty in bringing up his illness, how much the decision to move forward in our relationship had cost me, and how happy I was that I had followed the force driving me toward him and toward what would become the deepest love I had ever experienced.

The kids sat with me until Julian went out of the room and came back with a picture of us as a family. He put it on the table. Clarita imitated him and soon they had decorated the whole table with Morgan's tennis trophies, drawings they had done, more pictures.

"Daddy liked this," they said.

Both also wanted to remember their daddy with anecdotes: that Morgan liked sweets as much as they did and "stole" their chocolates. That if they woke in the middle of the night and Morgan was still awake watching news or sports, he would switch to cartoons and let them stay up with him for a bit instead of sending them back to bed.

The atmosphere was intimate but not solemn. We played a video with photos and music, which Cecilia, our best Uruguayan friend, had put together. We even laughed. Someone recounted the arguments Morgan and I had had at the beginning of our relationship. Mike remembered how Morgan managed to get everyone to like him. He recalled a trip to France where Morgan, at a very fine meal, had drunk Coca Cola straight from the bottle and a friend's father, the host of the meal, laughingly said he wouldn't forgive his own son for such bad manners—but he did forgive Morgan. Mike was right. I don't know how Morgan did it, but nothing he said went down wrong, ever.

The last one to speak, or try to speak, was Tamara via Skype. When I asked her if she wanted to say a few words, she burst into tears.

Three hours later the ceremony was over and the snowfall had turned into another massive storm. Nelson, Teresa, and her husband barely made it out of the city before they closed the airport, which would remain closed for three straight days. Outside was raw, but inside the house the warmth of all of us who loved Morgan continued to hang in the air, bringing me peace.

* * *

My cousin and his wife stayed with us for four more days and supported me while I received social calls. It all still felt surreal. The neighbors came in groups; I served them tea and cookies. I went to the office to say goodbye to colleagues, since I had already decided that I would travel to Argentina with the kids and we would stay through the end of February. A friend had booked us tickets for January 28.

I couldn't wait to be on that plane with Julian and Clarita, to go away for a while. I wanted to be nourished by my family, to feel their warmth, to be all together, to be helped with the kids. I could not stay at home, in that harsh winter. I needed to distance myself from Morgan's death in order to accept it, to gather strength before returning to Washington, DC, to a life that, I knew, would be totally new.

CHAPTER TEN

Another Life

I walked along the beach of Monte Hermoso and stopped near the lighthouse to write his name in the sand: Morgan. Five thousand miles from our shared home, under the sun and heat of the beaches of my childhood, the sensation of his death was, if possible, even more unreal. I was suspended between what had been and what was about to be. The calm clouds and steady lighthouse hinted that I too would someday feel steady again.

Both the kids and I felt comforted to be reunited with my mom and sister, and my brother-in-law and little niece. We needed this month to be with family. It had been such a long, excruciating process since we had been told that Morgan had six months to live . . . and my eight years with him had been so intense and so short. Now another stage was beginning. I couldn't yet face it head on.

Kiran, my best friend, flew in from Boston and met us at the airport when we returned to DC. She stayed with us for a week to cushion the shock of returning to a house without Morgan. The basement still held his bed and armchair. His belongings, books and photos were in every drawer of the house. I dreaded all the paperwork and bureaucracy that awaited me. To the rest of the world, I had a new status to declare: I was a widow.

As long as Morgan was alive, I had had incredible strength and energy. Adrenaline played a role, as my therapist had cautioned me, but I think my strength also came from the beginning of our relationship, when I had to decide whether or not to go forward with Morgan. I processed and accepted the possibility of the tumor's return early on, which helped me never think *why did this happen, we didn't deserve it, it's unfair.* Of course Morgan didn't deserve it, but I would deal with the reality in front of us, as painful as it was.

The hardest nights were yet to come, however. Kiran's support was the beginning of a year where I needed absolutely everyone around us, family and friends, neighbors and acquaintances, to help us begin the new life that awaited us.

* * *

One of the first things I had to do was to disassemble the room in the basement. Hospice services came to get the bed, but I had to decide where to put Morgan's chair, as well as safely dispose of the most dangerous medications myself. The carpet needed to be replaced. I wanted to turn the room into a pleasant, fresh space, both because we passed through it every day going into and out of the garage and because I wanted it to be a nice place for the kids to play as they grew up.

We reorganized and redecorated the living room and master bedroom, too. "Mommy, our house is like a beautiful hotel!" Julian exclaimed when all the work was done.

Little by little, the basement became a room where the kids liked to spend time. Now, filled with their toys, it didn't look like a place where their dad died. Sometimes even I forget death was there, even though the walls still display some of the countless drawings the kids did for Morgan and a tennis trophy I put up so he would be surrounded by good memories. The room also holds the urn with some of his ashes.

* * *

Before Morgan died, we talked about what do with his ashes. I asked if he wanted to do something special. He told me he didn't care, I could do whatever I wanted. I originally planned to scatter them in three places important to us: in Washington, DC, in Argentina, and in California, his favorite place in the world.

On the Potomac River, five blocks from our house, there is a beautiful little island, accessible via a pedestrian bridge. We used to walk around the island with the kids. It was one of Morgan's favorite places, so it seemed like the ideal place for part of him to stay.

When I got the call from the cremation service letting me know the ashes were ready to be picked up, I was with the kids in Argentina. Our nanny had to pick them up. When I got home they were already there, in a cardboard urn with a picture of a sunset, which I had liked much more than the usual pots. I decided to leave the ashes in the basement room. It was too much for me and the kids to do anything with them immediately. I would wait for some special occasion to scatter them. Then we got used to them being part of the house.

* * *

January 20, 2017, the day of the first anniversary of Morgan's death, was a gray, cold day, typical of winter in this city. That morning I took the kids to breakfast at Brooklyn Bagels, a place Morgan loved. We watched a movie at home. In the afternoon Phil and his wife came over. All together we wrote messages and drew pictures for Morgan on sheets of paper and folded them into boats. We went to the island in the Potomac River overlooking Georgetown. My usual route to work passes in front of that island, so I would see every day the place we scattered half of Morgan's ashes.

We tossed the little boats into the partly frozen river along with some candles and flowers. Remembering how much Morgan loved sweets, Phil added a chocolate to one. It was a ceremony similar to those performed on the Day of the Dead in Mexico, where people who have passed on are given an offering of their favorite things. Months later, the children's movie *Coco* was released, which portrays a boy on a journey to the world of the dead and underscores how memories keep the dead present to the living. The only question that Julian and Clarita asked when they saw it was how the main character had entered the world of the dead. I had been telling them since Morgan died that he is now a star in the sky, that he is looking at us and talking to our hearts. That day I felt that he was very, very close to us. We took pictures and silently watched the little boats leave.

The ashes did not fly away as I expected. Heavy, they fell at the water's edge, on the roots of the tree where I had perched to throw them. I felt that they were going to nourish it, that the cycle of life was continuing its course.

* * *

Four months after Morgan's death, Tamara passed away. I was devastated. We hadn't seen each other since before Morgan died because when we had the ceremony at home she was too sad, and too weak, to travel. Then I was trying to organize our life without Morgan and couldn't travel to Las Vegas to visit her. Her health got worse and worse. She moved into a friend's house in her last days, when her breast cancer metastasized to her ovaries. It was very hard for me and the kids to lose Tamara, especially so close to Morgan's death and from the same disease. They adored their grandmother. I loved her dearly too. She was very close to us. I miss not having her around, consulting her about things, asking her questions about Morgan.

Her death also reignited my concerns about a cancer trend in Morgan's family. I had already spoken to Dr. Gokaslan many times on behalf of my children. While the cancer that Morgan had suffered from was aggressive—it was only after his death that I learned the ependymoma had taken over everything, both the internal and external parts of his spine and sacrum—it had no genetic predisposition. However, between Tamara's death and Nelson's lymphoma, my fear returned and I asked the doctor one more time. He definitively reassured me that my kids were at no abnormally increased risk.

I was also worried that Julian and Clarita might think everyone was under the threat of cancer. For this reason, they kept going to art therapy, and together we all continued the therapy we started when I found out Morgan would die. We needed help through the mourning. I continued with my own psychologist and went to Life With Cancer for counseling and workshops at on relaxation and on paperwork and finances. Life With Cancer was a place of support for the whole family during those hard months, that first year which, in hindsight, went by like a blur, me busy with so much paperwork and with so many dear people around to cushion the huge blow we had just suffered.

I thought the first year after Morgan's death would be the worst of my life—and in many ways it was—but I barely had time to wallow in sadness. I had a family to raise. And a life to organize, from taking Morgan's name off the electric bill to figuring out what to do with his clothes, to managing bank accounts and tax returns . . . I remember words from *Memoirs of a Widow*, the extraordinary book that Joyce Carol Oates wrote after her husband's death: "The widow is someone who has discovered that there is no other choice," she says. And also, "Keep moving! That is salvation."

* * *

After Morgan's death I quickly noticed, at work and in general, that there started to be a little more perspective in my life. Things that maybe I used to worry about a lot or be very nervous about simply didn't matter as much anymore. Work had been my refuge during Morgan's illness and it was still my refuge now, during the bereavement.

I received a lot of support from my coworkers. Work has always been a place where I feel good, cheerful, proactive, and capable. It was comforting to have the office highlight my strengths. That type of soft cushion that people form around you is something that is lost over time, when one returns from the category of "widow" to the category of "normal person."

I went back to work travel: Kenya, China, Korea, Tunisia, Nepal, Uganda. A question that I had never thought of before arose before each trip: what if something happens to me? Maria, our nanny, was designated as responsible for Julian and Clarita—a temporary guardian only when I was traveling—with a team of neighbors and friends who could give her a hand if she needed it. That had not happened before. I had to draw up all the papers stipulating with whom the children would stay if a misfortune were to happen to me. I decided that it would be my sister Virginia and her family, and if she couldn't take care of them, it would be Teresa, my sister-in-law. All this made the decision to travel at all more difficult.

Although I knew that the most important thing that first year was to adapt to the new situation without making rash decisions, I could not avoid the questions: would it be better to move to a smaller house? Would it be a good idea to go back to Argentina, to be close to my family? Did I need a quieter job? What made the most sense for me, for my children?

* * *

I actually enjoyed sorting and classifying Morgan's belongings: going through his CDs, for example, hearing in my head the music he liked. I looked one more time at all the photos he had taken, the huge collection he had stored in a closet in the garage. I rearranged his books as well.

I did part with his clothes soon after his death. I asked Nelson, Teresa, and his friends Phil and Mike if they wanted to keep anything. Nelson took some t-shirts, a jacket, and stuff from Morgan's bike. Phil took a shirt, Mike another item. Teresa took a tie and a t-shirt.

Morgan had a wonderful collection of button-down shirts, and I asked an Argentinian friend who sews beautiful quilts to make one for Julian and one for

Clarita. We managed to meet in New York and I took all the shirts to her. She sent me some possible patterns and each of the kids chose one. Clarita gravitated toward a star pattern featuring all different colors. Julian chose a more geometric one, with gradient colors toward the ends. Both quilts have a geometric patchwork on the back. Their dad's shirts are now works of art, warm and handmade, which they use as bed blankets.

I donated Morgan's jackets and shoes, but I kept his glasses and glasses holder. Sometimes I take them out and look at them with the kids. I think they might want to have them in the future. They already play games on some of his old cell phones. While I don't need anything special to bring him to mind, sometimes I choose to remember by putting on "And Now You're Leaving," a song about separation with lyrics referencing a last breath. I listened to it often on my trips to Baltimore when Morgan was a patient there. It's a song that makes me cry inconsolably and I weep alone in my room listening to it, hugging a fluffy sweater that is perhaps my favorite of Morgan's belongings.

I also started actually using things we had kept in storage before. For example, the beautiful china that Tamara gave us now sits in an accessible glass cabinet. I bring it out frequently when we have friends over for dinner. I feel that, by using it, I am honoring not only Morgan but also his mom and our life as a family.

* * *

A few months after Morgan's death, I got in touch again with Diego, my old boyfriend from Bahía Blanca. We talked on the phone; he was also going through a difficult family moment. We still have a lot of affection for each other and we connected through daily calls for a while. In my diary I wrote something that sums up my first year without Morgan: "I need a hug." And while it was nice to think about Diego and be in touch with him, I never thought it was his hug that I needed.

On our annual vacation in Monte Hermoso, my mom, sister and I have a ritual: to take stock of the year that is ending, to think about what we would like to do or achieve in the year that is beginning. As 2016 turned to 2017 I realized that, though the gold wedding ring was still shining on my finger, I hadn't truly been married for a year.

I think it took me that whole year to start my life again. In January 2017, after the anniversary of Morgan's death and the scattering of his ashes, I realized that I was finally almost done with the multiplicity of paperwork I had to do. For the rest of the world I was back to being the same old Laura, and the "recent widow" sign was no longer hanging over my head. It struck me anew that this was my everyday life, that Morgan was really gone, and gone forever.

I decided to take off my ring and put it away. I knew I was going to miss it. I had loved looking at it, feeling it on my hand, the way it looked on me. But it was no longer realistic to have it on. When we landed back in DC from Argentina, it was a shock that no one was waiting for us at the airport. That also marked a new beginning.

I placed the wedding band in my jewelry box, next to Morgan's.

*   *   *

Adjusting to Morgan's absence required something different month after month. The kids, the house, the job, everything was a huge responsibility for me. It was impossible to feel as light as I did before the illness broke into our lives.

In July 2017, the kids and I went to a resort in Mexico that offered separate activities for each of us. I joined in a card game with other guests. Maybe it was being around strangers or being in an unfamiliar place, but it was one of the first times after all we had been through where I felt quiet settle inside me. I really relaxed. The kids played with other kids and I fully enjoyed myself for the first time in a long time. After that trip, pleasure arose more and more frequently. With time, which shapes everything and calms everything, I was able to get back to feeling happy about the good things I still had in my life.

I read *Option B*, the book Sheryl Sandberg, COO of Facebook, wrote after her husband died suddenly of a heart attack. In her previous book, *Lean In*, she talked about the importance of sharing family tasks with a husband so that a woman can really take advantage of job opportunities, to break the famous "glass ceiling." When I read it in the midst of Morgan's illness, I thought: *What about those of us who have a sick husband?* In this new book, Sandberg realized how difficult it all is for a woman who has to run a household and raise children alone. For those of us who had an Option A of partner support, Option B means doing the best we can with what we have now.

I also saw my experience reflected in Sandberg's observation that many people are uncomfortable talking about the person who died. Sandberg describes a dinner party where everyone was sharing how they had met their partners. Perhaps believing it was disrespectful or insensitive to ask, they skipped her. She says that, on the contrary, she wants to keep talking about her husband, such an important part of her life, even though he is no longer here. It's the same for me. I still feel I need to talk about Morgan, to express myself, sadly or not. We had a wonderful love story. Meeting him was so important and our eight years of love were so beautiful and meaningful. And our children are my pride.

A few months after Morgan died, on a plane to Kenya for a business trip, I thought about how I didn't want to forget anything, absolutely anything about our relationship. As if somehow—again I'm reminded of *Coco*, the children's movie—if I remembered exactly how everything happened over the years, Morgan would still remain with us, bound by that memory. I thought it was important for the kids to have a written testimony. Plus, I have always loved biographies and autobiographies.

Our story was short—very short—but we lived it intensely. And it is worth telling. Those ideas led me to write this book.

*   *   *

I asked for memories of Morgan from his sister, from his father, and from Phil and Mike. I wanted to incorporate all of their impressions of and feelings about Morgan. In one email, Nelson told me:

> I would like to add, regarding Morgan, that he meant much more to me than the sum of the stories I have told you. I loved being around him. It felt great to be in his presence. It may sound strange but I loved seeing him in motion. I loved his energy. The best thing was traveling with him, spending time by his side. Besides being smart, he was never in a bad mood. He loved to laugh and liked me to repeat over and over quotes or lines from movie scenes that we thought were funny. I think about him every day. Some mornings, I wake up reliving the bad times of his illness. How did we survive that? Well, I wanted to add these words. I miss you guys, see you soon. Hopefully Julian will play in Little League, so that part of Morgan lives on. Be well, Nelson.

*   *   *

Julian and Clarita, like Morgan's family, like myself, also lived—and still live—their own process. They have gone through things too overwhelming for their age.

We continue to do family grief therapy, playing games that bring up death and memories, finding ways they can integrate what happened to us into their lives, that they can talk about it. One game centered on questions like, "When someone dies, can they live again?" Clarita quickly answered no.

"And why?" asked the therapist.

"Because there is the skeleton and there is nothing there." Clarita has no problem talking about the subject, she does it very naturally.

Julian is the shyest. He prefers not to talk about Morgan in front of other people, only with his sister and me. It is generally difficult for him to express his feelings. Not long ago he hugged me and started crying, telling me that he missed Daddy, that he was afraid of forgetting him. In front of others, his attitude is different. He sometimes talks about Morgan in the present tense without realizing it, as I do, too: "my daddy is a lawyer," or "my parents are at home."

Last Father's Day, Julian's school had the kids do some dad-related activities. I had gone to talk to the teacher and request that he be careful with the subject. When I saw that they asked the children how old is your dad, what color are his eyes, what are his hobbies . . . it made my heart ache. They continued the theme the following day, making it even more painful for Julian. For several days he cried over anything and nothing. But I knew the real source of the tears.

There isn't a day that goes by that Clara doesn't talk about Morgan: "I miss Daddy. I love Daddy. Daddy is a star now, I carry him in my heart." She also makes up songs about how her daddy and grandmother died and are together in heaven. One day at the supermarket she saw a picture of the four of us together that I have in my wallet and she asked to hold it while I was looking for something in a gondola. I saw that she was moving it.

"What are you doing with the picture, Clarita?"

"I'm showing it to Daddy."

It is important to me, especially now, that they both feel close to their paternal family, even though they live far away. I decided that we would make a new tradition of celebrating Thanksgiving in Phoenix with Teresa and her family. On the last trip, Julian and his cousin Nate didn't leave each other's side for a moment. They played and slept in the same room for four days straight.

I like that my children have family traditions. Even though neither Morgan nor I were practicing our respective religions, I would like Julian and Clara to continue to keep some of the Jewish customs from their father's side, just so they know their heritage, and to observe the traditional Argentine Catholic holidays of Christmas and Easter.

We always talk about Morgan in a happy way. I always bring him up, so they don't forget their dad. Father's Day, Morgan's birthday, the anniversary of his death . . . these are days where I like to take them to do things Morgan enjoyed. Having bagels for breakfast, going to Barnes & Noble, going to the movies, crossing to the island at sunset, when the pink glow of the sky reflects on the Potomac River, to see "our" tree . . . these are little rituals to honor and remember him.

Of course, I don't always know the best way to accompany them on this path. Their reactions can take me by surprise. Like the day when Julian asked me why this had happened to us, and I didn't know how to answer him other than to hug him tightly and tell him that I was sad too, and that it was okay to feel that way. Or when I showed them the video of Morgan reading the stories he had recorded for them during his days in the basement room and the kids were shocked to see their dad on screen. It confused and sensitized them.

It's hard being alone to raise them. It's hard sometimes to know whether I'm doing things right with them. Not having Morgan's advice, his parenting support, his common sense, being unable to call him multiple times a day to consult on some decision concerning the kids . . . I miss that pillar terribly. That, and his loving way of talking to me, are perhaps the things I miss most about my husband.

* * *

I recently had to fill out a form asking for an emergency contact. It is not the first form I have filled out asking for this kind of information, but this time it jolted me. What am I doing here in the United States if I am alone? I don't have a good emergency contact! It is my nanny! My mom is in Bahía Blanca, my sister is in Mendoza; I don't have someone in Washington,

DC who is as unconditional as they are. I thought maybe I should go back to Argentina. It was a powerful moment.

I realize that, now in the third year after Morgan's death, I have the tools to move forward. I am steadier, I no longer consult a psychologist or a coach. I am more focused on my work and my career as a senior economist. I feel strong and happy. And ready for new adventures, new paths: in August 2018, I will move with Julian and Clarita for three years to Cairo!

I was offered a promotion in my job: leading the human capital program based in the capital of Egypt. An amazing work schedule, full of new challenges. We will live in a beautiful place, the kids will go to an American school. And a friend from Washington, DC, by chance, will also move to the same city. It didn't take me long to decide. I feel that the three of us deserved a new adventure, now that we are strong and united, and that Morgan, wherever he is, is supporting us. Like a flower peeking timidly in the first months of thaw, I feel happy again with the kids, with my house, with my family, my friends, my new job. My memories. And I hope that, in the future, I may even fall in love again. I am still the romantic I always was.

* * *

It comforts me to think that Morgan, despite dying so young, had a happy life. When I knew him, he had already had the early operations, which had greatly limited him in the physical activity he loved, in travel, in social life and sports, all things that had been central to his life up to that point. However, I know that he was satisfied with what he had done in life. Of course, Julian and Clarita were his greatest pride and source of happiness. I think his sense of accomplishment helped him to handle the cancer and all the bad things the cancer brought to us with dignity and tenacity.

I still feel him by my side. He's in the picture of the four of us on the beach in New Jersey that I have on my desk at work. In the silent conversations I sometimes have with him, as if he is indeed the star that I and Julian and Clarita say he is, and he is listening to me from somewhere up there. On his side of the bed, where I still stretch my hand between dreams and wonder where he is. In those same dreams.

I still have fresh in my mind, as if it were today, the moment I decided to stay by Morgan's side. When we barely knew each other, for all the good and all the bad. When illness was a possibility that dyed our horizon black but, at the same time, seemed so unlikely. Is it a story that ended badly? I can't look at it that way. Sometimes I cry when I think about it. But I cry with a full spectrum of emotion: I knew exactly what the consequences could be, and it still seems to me, even as I bring this book to a close and open a new chapter in my life, that it was the best decision I ever made.

Made in the USA
Monee, IL
04 November 2026

67380068R00098